The Easy Cookbook for

Keto Diet

The Complete Guide to Lose Weight More Easily and Change Your Lifestyle Without Suffering. Breakfast, Lunch and Dinner Recipes.

Angela D. Cook

before attempting any techniques outlined in this book. By reading this document, the reader agrees that under no circumstances are the author responsible for any losses, direct or indirect, which are incurred due to the use of information within this document, including, but not limited to, errors, omissions, or inaccuracies.

Contents

Chapter 1: Breakfast recipes

PANCAKES

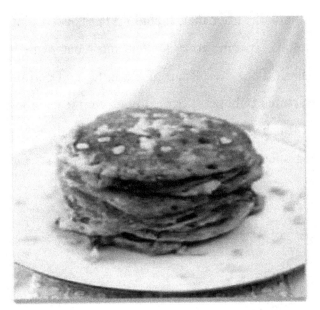

Ingredients

- 1 or 2 cups flour
- 1 tablespoonful baking powder
- 1/2 tablespoonful kosher salt
- 1/4 tablespoonful ground ginger

- 1/4 tablespoonful pumpkin pie spice
- 1/3 cup maple syrup
- 2/4 cup water Mix
- 1/4 cup + 1 tablespoonful crystallized ginger slices together.

Instructions:

In a neat bowl, mix together the first five recipes. Add flour with syrup with water and stir; after that, including the hacked ginger and mix until-just-joined—warm your skillet and coat with a non-stick cooking splash. Pour in 1/4 cup of the hitter and permit it to warm until it structures bubbles. Permit to cook until caramelized. Serve warm and finished off with a slathering of vegetarian spread, a sprinkle of maple syrup, and decorated with slashed sweetened ginger.

Wholesome Facts

Servings per holder 4

Prep Total 10 min

Serving Size 2/3 cup (20g)

Sum per serving Calories 20 % Daily Value Total Facts 10g 10% Saturated Fat 0g 7% Trans Fat 2g - Cholesterol 3% Sodium 10mg 2% Total Carbohydrate 7g 3% Dietary Fiber 2g 4% Total Sugar 1g - Protein 3gVitamin C 2mcg 10% Calcium 260mg 20% Iron 8mg 30% Potassium 235mg 6%

Chinese-Style Zucchini with Ginger

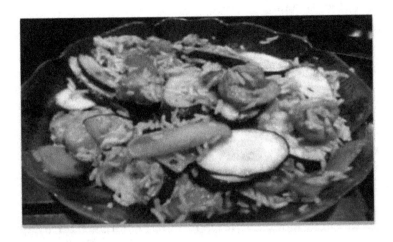

Ingredients

1 teaspoon oil

1 lb. zucchini cut into

1/4-inch slices

1/2 cup vegetarian broth

2 teaspoons light soy sauce

1 teaspoon dry sherry

1 teaspoon toasted sesame oil

Instructions:

Warmth an enormous wok or hefty skillet over high heat until hot at that point, add the oil. In the end, when the oil is hot, add the zucchini and ginger—sautéed food one moment. Add the stock, soy sauce, and sherry. Sautéed food over high warmth until the store cooks down a piece and the zucchini is fresh delicate. Eliminate from the heat, sprinkle with sesame oil and serve.

Wholesome Facts

Servings per holder 10

Prep Total 10 min

Serving Size 2/3 cup (55g)

Sum per serving Calories 20 % Daily Value Total Fat 8g 6% Saturated Fat 1g 2% Trans Fat 0g - Cholesterol 0% Sodium 160mg 9% Total Carbohydrate 37g 50%Dietary Fiber 4g 2 Total Sugar 12g - Protein 3g Vitamin C 2mcg 1% Calcium 260mg 8% Iron 8mg 17% Potassium 235mg 8%

Breakfast Super Antioxidant Berry Smoothie

Ingredients 1 cup of filtered water 1 whole orange, peeled, de-seeded & cut into chunks 2 cups frozen raspberries or blackberries 1 Tablespoon goji berries 1 1/2 Tablespoons hemp seeds or plant-based protein powder 2 cups leafy greens (parsley, spinach, or kale) Instructions: Blend on high until smooth Serve and drink immediately.

Nutritional Facts Servings per container 5 Prep Total 10 min Serving Size 4 cup (20g) Amount per serving Calories 20 % Daily Value Total Fat 2g 5% Saturated Fat 2g 4% Trans Fat 7g - Cholesterol 2% Sodium 7mg 9% Total Carbohydrate 20g 20% Dietary Fiber 4g 20%Total

Sugar 12g - Protein 3g Vitamin C 2mcg 15% Calcium 260mg 7% Iron 8mg 4% Potassium 235mg 1%

Cucumber Tomato Surprise

Ingredients Chopped 1 medium of tomato 1 small cucumber peeled in stripes and chopped 1 large avocado cut into cubes 1 half of a lemon or lime squeezed ½ tsp. Himalayan or Real salt 1 Teaspoon of original olive oil, MCT or coconut oil.

Instructions: Mix everything together and enjoy. This dish tastes even better after sitting for 40 – 60 minutes. Blend into a soup if desired.

Nutritional Facts Servings per container 5 Prep Total 10 min Serving Size 2/3 cup (55g) Amount per serving Calories 2 % Daily Value Total Fat 20g 17% Saturated Fat 2g 1% Trans Fat 1.2g - Cholesterol 20% Sodium 55mg 12% Total Carbohydrate 14g 50% Dietary Fiber 4g 8%Total Sugar 2g - Protein 7g Vitamin C 2mcg 10% Calcium 20mg 2% Iron 1mg 5% Potassium 210mg 7%

Chewy Chocolate Chip Cookies

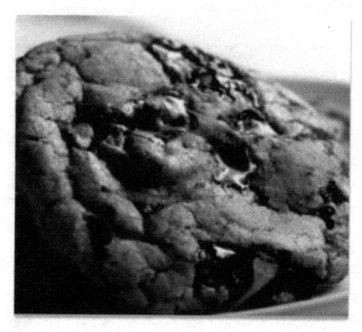

Ingredients

1 cup veggie-lover margarine, relaxed ½ cup white sugar ½ cup earthy colored sugar ¼ cup sans dairy milk 1 teaspoon vanilla 2 ¼ cups flour ½ teaspoon salt 1 teaspoon heating soft drink 12 ounces sans dairy chocolate chips

Instructions:

Preheat broiler to 350°F. In a large bowl, blend the spread, white sugar, and earthy colored sugar until light and relaxing. Gradually mix in the sans dairy milk and afterward add the vanilla to make a velvety blend. In a different bowl, join the flour, salt, and heating pop. You need to add this dry blend to the fluid combination and mix it well—

crease in the chocolate chips. Drop a little spoonful of the player onto non-stick treat sheets and heat for 9 minutes.

Healthful Facts Servings per holder 10 Prep Total 10 min Serving Size 2/3 cup (40g) Amount per serving Calories 10 % Daily Value Total Fat 10g 2% Saturated Fat 1g 5% Trans Fat 0g - Cholesterol 15% Sodium 120mg 8% Total Carbohydrate 21g 10% Dietary Fiber 4g 1%Total Sugar 1g 0% Protein 6g Vitamin C 2mcg 7% Calcium 210mg 51% Iron 8mg 1% Potassium 235mg 10%

Benedict Eggs

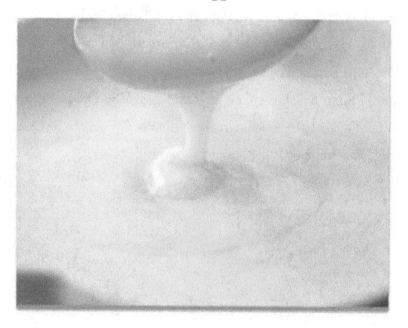

TIME: 20 MINUTES

Nutritional Facts Calories: 624 Total fat: 53.9g Carbohydrates: 1.8g Net carbohydrates 1.8g Fiber: 0g Protein: 32.6g

Ingredients

FOR THE HOLLANDAISE SAUCE

2 eggs 1 1/2 teaspoons freshly squeezed lemon juice 1/4 cup butter, melted 1/4 teaspoon salt

FOR THE EGGS

4 slices of bacon 1 teaspoon of vinegar 4 eggs

Preparation

Make the hollandaise sauce In a large bowl, beat two eggs and the lemon juice together vigorously until you get a solid whole and almost double in volume. Fill a large frying pan with 2.5 cm of water and heat until it simmers. Reduce the heat to medium. Wear an oven glove and hold the bowl with the eggs above the water and make sure it does not touch the water. Beat the mixture for about 3 minutes and make sure you do not mix the eggs. Slowly add the butter to the egg mixture and keep beating until thick, about 2 minutes. Stir in the salt. Stir the sauce until it has cooled. Make the eggs. Pour the water from the pan and place it over medium heat. Place the bacon in the pan—Bake for 3 minutes per side. Transfer the bacon onto paper towels. Add the vinegar and apply over low heat to a medium-sized pan, half-full of water.

To serve

Break bacon in half. Place two halves on a plate and garnish with an egg. Repeat with 2 more halves and another egg. Cover with hollandaise sauce. Repeat with the remaining bacon and the eggs for the second portion.

Scottish Eggs

TIME: 45 MINUTES

Nutritional Facts

Calories: 258 Total fat: 20.5g Carbohydrates: 14.2g Net carbohydrates 1g Fiber: 0g Protein: 16.7g

Ingredients

1⁄2 cup breakfast frankfurter 1⁄2 teaspoon garlic powder 1/4 teaspoon salt 1⁄8 teaspoon newly ground dark pepper 2 hard-bubbled eggs, stripped.

Planning

Preheat the broiler to 200 ° C. Blend the frankfurter, garlic powder, salt, and pepper in a medium bowl. Shape the wiener into two balls—smooth each ball on a piece of heating paper into a 0.8 cm thick baked good. Spot a hard-bubbled egg in the focal point of every pie and cautiously shape the hotdog around the egg. Spot the frankfurter-covered eggs on a non-lubed heating sheet and spot them in the preheated broiler. Prepare for 25 minutes. Permit to cool for 5 minutes and serve. EXTRA: Breakfast wiener is a regular American sort of pork hotdog, and you can utilize something like frankfurters.

Biscuits in Sausage gravy

TIME: 50 MINUTES

Nutritional Facts

Calories: 559 Total fat: 48.5g Carbohydrates: 14.2g Net carbohydrates 8.2g Fiber: 6g Protein: 14.6g

Ingredients

FOR THE Biscuits

1/2 cup coconut flour

1/2 cup almond flour

2 teaspoons baking powder

1 teaspoon garlic powder

1/2 teaspoon onion powder

1/2 teaspoon salt

1/2 cup grated Cheddar cheese.

1/4 cup butter, melted.

4 eggs

3/4 cup sour cream

For SAUSAGE Gravy

450 grams ground breakfast wiener 1 teaspoon finely hacked garlic 1 tablespoon almond flour 1 1/2 cup unsweetened almond milk 1/2 cup hefty (whipped) cream 1 1/2 teaspoon newly ground dark pepper 1/2 teaspoon salt

Readiness

Preheat the broiler to 180 ° C Cover a preparing sheet with heating paper. In an enormous bowl, blend coconut flour, almond flour, heating powder, garlic powder, onion powder, and salt. Gradually mix in the cheddar. Make a pit in the dry fixings before adding the wet fixings. Add the dissolved spread, eggs, and sharp cream to this pit. Overlap together until the mixture is shaped. Utilize a spoon to drop rolls onto the readied preparing sheet, place them 2.5 cm apart. Bake the treats for 20 minutes or until they are firm and light earthy colored.

Arrangement of the wiener sauce

Warmth a huge container over medium warmth. Add the ground wiener, open it with a spoon, and heat it earthy colored on all sides. Add the cleaved garlic when the wiener is earthy colored—Cook for 1 moment. On the off chance that the garlic is fragrant, sprinkle the almond flour over it. Turn the warmth low to medium-low. Permit the almond flour to mix into the fat to build up a light roux, blending continually, for around 5 minutes. Gradually add the almond milk to the roux, mixing constantly. Add the whipped cream. Increment the temperature to medium-high, mix and decrease the combination for 3 minutes. Turn the warmth to low to medium-low. Add the pepper and salt. Mix for 1 moment. Check the rolls and eliminate the preparing sheet from the stove when you're set. Allow the bread rolls to cool for 5 minutes. Decrease the warmth again under the wiener sauce to low. Stew while the bread rolls cool. When the bread rolls cool, serve 1 for every individual and embellishment with a ⅓ cup of sauce.

Portobello, Sausage, and Cheese "Breakfast Burger"

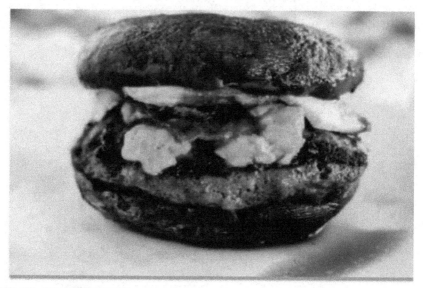

TIME: 25 MINUTES

Nutritional Facts

Calories: 504 Total fat: 41.1g Carbohydrates: 10.1g Net carbohydrates 7g Fiber: 3.1g Protein: 23.8g

Ingredients

1 tablespoon olive oil 2 Portobello mushrooms, stalk removed1/4 cup breakfast sausage 2 (50 grams) slices of Cheddar cheese

Preparation

Heat the olive oil for 1 minute in a medium-sized non-stick frying pan over medium heat. Place the mushrooms in the hot oil, with the convex side up. Bake for about 5 minutes per side or until browned.

Heat another medium-sized frying pan over medium heat. Form the breakfast sausage into a 1 cm thick pastry. Place it in the center of the heated pan—Bake for 4 to 5 minutes. Turn and bake for another 2 to 3 minutes. When the sausage is almost ready, turn down the heat. Garnish the burger with Cheddar cheese. Cook until the cheese melts. Transfer the mushrooms from the skillet to a plate. Place the cheese-covered pie on one mushroom. Cover with the remaining mushroom cap and serve.

Cinnamon Muffins with Butter Frosting

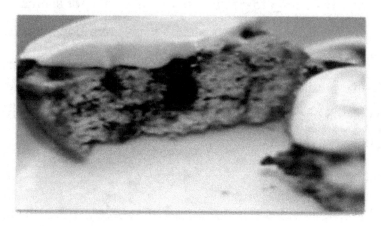

TIME: 50 MINUTES

Nutritional Facts

Calories: 225 Total fat: 18.5g Carbohydrates: 6.2g Net carbohydrates 3.1g Fiber: 3.1g Protein: 5.3g

Ingredients

FOR CINNAMON MUFFINS

1 cup almond flour 1/2 cup coconut flour 2 teaspoons baking powder 1/4 cup erythritol or another sugar substitute, such as stevia 6 eggs 1/2 cup butter, melted 1/2 cup sparkling water 1 teaspoon pure vanilla extract 1 1/2 tablespoons cinnamon.

FOR ICE CREAM

Glaze 1 pack of cream cheese, at room temperature 1 tablespoon of sour cream 1/2 teaspoon of pure vanilla extract

Preparation of muffins

Preheat the oven to 180 ° C. In a medium bowl, beat together the almond flour, coconut flour, baking powder, and erythritol. Beat the eggs in a large bowl. Add the melted butter, sparkling water, and vanilla. Beat to combine. Add the dry ingredients to the wet ingredients. Mix well. Put the batter evenly in a frying pan. Garnish each muffin with an equal amount of cinnamon. Stir the cinnamon through the batter with a toothpick. Place the cup form in the preheated oven—Bake for 20 to 25 minutes or until golden brown. Remove the pan from the oven and cool the muffins in the pan for 5 to 10 minutes.

Preparation of the Cream Cheese Glaze

In a medium bowl, mix cream cheese, sour cream, and vanilla. Cool until needed. Spread evenly over the muffins before serving.

Almond Flour Pancakes

TIME: 35 MINUTES

Nutritional Facts

Calories: 383 Total fat: 34g Carbohydrates: 7.9g Net carbohydrates 3.9g Fiber: 4g Protein: 3.8g

Ingredients

1 cup almond flour

1 tablespoon stevia or another sugar substitute

1/4 teaspoon salt

1 teaspoon baking powder2 eggs

1⁄8 cup heavy (whipped) cream

1⁄8 cup sparkling water.

1⁄2 teaspoon pure vanilla extract

2 tablespoons coconut oil, melted Baking spray for grill plate (plancha)

Preparation

Heat a grill plate over medium heat. In a large bowl, mix almond flour, stevia, salt, and baking powder. Make a small hole in the middle of the dry ingredients. Add the eggs, heavy cream, sparkling water, vanilla, and coconut oil. Mix everything well. Spray the grill plate with baking spray. Pour the batter into the desired quantities on the grill plate. Bake the pancakes for 2 to 3 minutes until you see tiny bubbles and then turn over—Bake for 1 to 2 minutes. Remove the pancakes from the baking sheet when they are ready. Repeat with the remaining batter.

Raspberry Scones

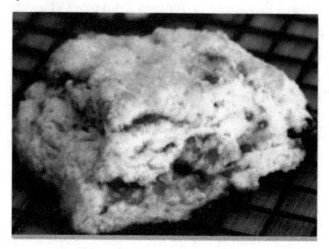

TIME: 35 MINUTES

Nutritional Facts

Calories: 133 Total fat: 8.6g Carbohydrates: 4g Net carbohydrates 2g
Fiber: 2g Protein: 1.5g

Ingredients

1 cup almond flour 2 eggs, beaten 1/3 cup Splenda, stevia, or another
sugar substitute 1 1/2 teaspoon pure vanilla extract1 1/2 teaspoon
baking powder 1/2 cup raspberries.

Preparation

Preheat the broiler to 180 ° C. Cover a preparing sheet with heating
paper. In a considerable bowl, blend almond flour, eggs, Splenda,

vanilla, and heating powder. Blend well. Add the raspberries to the bowl and overlay them incautiously. After the raspberries have been prepared, scoop 2 to 3 tablespoons of player, per scone, onto the heating plate fixed with composing the paper. Spot the preparing plate in the preheated stove. Prepare for 15 minutes or until light earthy colored. Eliminate the preparing sheet from the broiler. Spot the scones on a rack to cool for 10 minutes.

INGREDIENT TIP:

Depending on the raspberries' size, you can cut the raspberries into two halves before adding them to the batter. By doing this, the raspberry flavor is spread over the entire scone.

Waffles with whipped cream

TIME: 15 MINUTES

Nutritional Facts

Calories: 420 Total fat: 27.1g Carbohydrates: 15.7g Net carbohydrates: 6.5g Fiber: 9.2g Protein: 27g

Ingredients

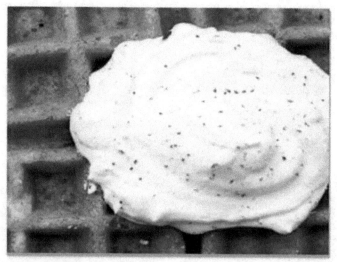

FOR THE WAFFLES

Baking spray for waffle iron 1/4 cup coconut flour 1/4 cup almond flour 1/4 cup flax flour 1 teaspoon baking powder 1 teaspoon stevia or another sugar substitute 1/4 teaspoon cinnamon 3/4 cup protein (about 3 proteins) 4 eggs 1 teaspoon pure vanilla extract

FOR THE WHIP CREAM

1/2 cup of heavy (whipped) cream 1 teaspoon of stevia or another sugar substitute

Preparation

Prepare the waffles. Heat the waffle maker to medium height. Cover with baking spray. In a large bowl, beat together the coconut flour, almond flour, flax flour, baking powder, stevia, and cinnamon. Beat the egg whites in another medium-sized bowl until stiff peaks occur. Add the whole eggs and vanilla to the dry ingredients. Mix well. Carefully fold the whipped egg whites through the dry ingredients until completely absorbed. Pour the batter onto the preheated waffle maker. Bake according to the instructions of the waffle maker.

Prepare the whipped cream.

Beat the heavy cream in a medium bowl for 3 to 4 minutes until thick. Add the stevia. Continue to beat until stiff peaks form, about 1 minute. Garnish the waffles with equal amounts of whipped cream and serve.

Cream cheese pancakes

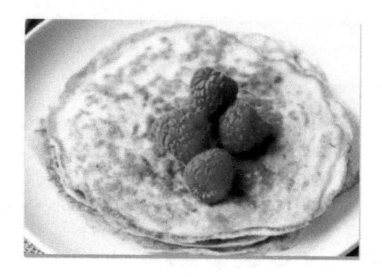

TIME: 15 MINUTES

Nutritional Facts

Calories: 327 Total fat: 28.7g Carbohydrates: 2.5g Net carbohydrates: 2.5g Fiber: 0g Protein: 15.4g

Ingredients

1/4 cup cream cheese, at room temperature 2 eggs 1/2 teaspoon of stevia 1/4 teaspoon of nutmeg

Preparation

Heat a grill plate (plancha) over medium heat. Place the cream cheese in a blender. Add the eggs, stevia, and nutmeg. Mix until the batter is smooth. Slowly pour a small amount of batter onto the grill plate, about a one-eighth cup per pancake. The batter will be very thin and easy to spread. Bake the pancake a little longer than a minute before turning it over gently. Let it bake for another minute before you take it out of the pan. Repeat with the remaining batter.

Denver Omelet

TIME: 15 MINUTES

Nutritional Facts

Calories: 429 Total fat: 32.7g Carbohydrates: 9.1g Net carbohydrates: 6.9g Fiber: 2.2g Protein: 24.7g

Ingredients

1 tablespoon margarine 1/4 cup slashed onion 1/4 cup cleaved red pepper 1/4 cup hacked green pepper1/2 teaspoon slashed garlic 1/4 cup cooked ham, cubed 2 eggs, beaten 1/4 teaspoon salt 1/8 teaspoon newly ground dark pepper 1/4 cup ground cheddar.

Readiness

Dissolve the spread in a medium-sized non-stick skillet over medium warmth. Add the onion, red pepper, green pepper, garlic, and ham. Cook until the ham is firm, around 2 minutes. In a bit of a bowl, beat the eggs with salt and pepper. Empty the eggs into the container with the vegetables and the ham. Lessen the warmth to medium—Cook the eggs for 3 to 4 minutes. Turn the omelet. After pivoting, sprinkle the upper portion of the omelet with the cheddar. Following 1 or 2 minutes, overlap the omelet and cover the cheddar. Cook another 1 to 2 minutes until the cheddar dissolves. Eliminate the omelet from the container and serve.

AVOCADO EGG BOWLS

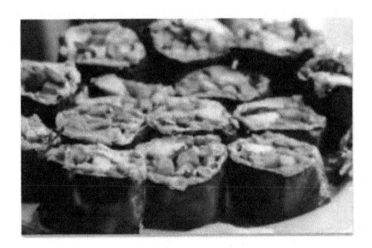

Ingredients

- 2 sheets of raw or toasted sushi nori
- 1 large Romaine leaf cut in half down the length of the spine.
- 2 Teaspoons of spicy miso paste
- 1 avocado peeled and sliced.
- ½ red, yellow, or orange bell pepper, julienned.
- ½ cucumber, peeled, seeded, and julienned.
- ½ cup raw sauerkraut
- ½ carrot, beet or zucchini, shredded.
- 1 cup alfalfa or favorite green sprouts
- 1 small bowl of water for sealing roll

Instructions:

Place a sheet of nori on a sushi rolling mat or washcloth, lining it up at the end closest to you. Place the Romaine leaf on the edge of the nori with the spine most intimate to you. Spread Spicy Miso Paste on the Romaine Line the plate with all ingredients in descending order, placing sprouts on last Roll the Nori sheet away from you, tucking the ingredients in with your fingers, and seal the roll with water or Spicy Miso Paste. Slice the roll into 6 or 8 rounds.

Nutritional Facts

Servings per container 10

Prep Total 10 min

Serving Size 2/3 cup (70g)

Amount per serving Calories 15 % Daily Value Total Fat 2g 10% Saturated Fat 1g 9% Trans Fat 10g - Cholesterol 1% Sodium 70mg 5% Total Carbohydrate 22g 40% Dietary Fiber 4g 2%Total Sugar 12g - Protein 3g Vitamin C 2mcg 2% Calcium 260mg 7% Iron 8mg 2% Potassium 235mg 4%

Chapter 2: LUNCH RECIPES

Cajun Grilled Chicken

PREP TIME: 30 MIN

COOK TIME: 15 MIN

YIELD: 2 SERVINGS

INGREDIENTS

½ teaspoon dried oregano ½ teaspoon dried thyme 1 teaspoon smoked or regular paprika ¼ teaspoon cayenne pepper 1 garlic clove, finely chopped 1 teaspoon canola oil Four 5-ounce skinless, boneless chicken breasts.

Bean salad

2 tomatoes, diced 2/3 cup frozen sweet corn, defrosted 1 cup canned black-eyed or cannellini beans, rinsed and drained 2 scallions, chopped ¼ cup sundried tomatoes Zest and juice of 1 lime 1 tablespoon fresh cilantro leaves, chopped.

Guacamole

1 ripe avocado ¼ teaspoon red chili pepper ½ tablespoon extra-virgin olive oil 1 lime, juiced 1 tablespoon fresh cilantro leaves, chopped.

DIRECTIONS

1 For the chicken flavoring, blend every one of the spices, flavors, finely cleaved garlic clove, and oil in a large plastic sack, add water to make the marinade more fluid. Spot a chicken bosom between two sheets of waxed material or transparent plastic film. Pound with a hammer or moving pin to smooth; transfer to the plastic sack and rehash with residual bosoms. Blend satisfactorily and seal. Put on the side pack to marinate for 15 minutes.

2 For the bean serving of mixed greens, de-seed and dice the tomatoes. Add to a huge blending bowl with the corn, beans, hacked scallions, finely cleaved sundried tomatoes, and cilantro. Zing the lime and afterward cut down the middle. Add the zing and juice of the lime and blend entirely into the plate of mixed greens.

3 For the guacamole, scoop and pit 1 entire avocado and pound to favored consistency. Add finely slashed bean stew pepper, olive oil, lime juice, and cilantro. Blend in by crushing with a fork. 4 Lightly oil barbecue surface and preheat flame broil to medium-high warmth. Spot chicken on the flame broil for 7 to 8 minutes. Flip over and cook an extra 7 to 8 minutes or until no remaining pink parts. Chicken arrives at 165 degrees F. Serve every chicken bosom on a plate with the bean plate of mixed greens and a scoop of guacamole.

PER SERVING: Calories 520; Total fat: 23g; Saturated fat: 3.5g; Cholesterol: 80mg; Sodium: 150mg; Carbohydrates: 42g; Fiber: 16g; Sugar: 10g; Protein: 45g

Honey-Crusted Salmon with Spinach

PREP TIME: 10 MIN

COOK TIME: 15 MIN

YIELD: 4 SERVINGS

INGREDIENTS

1½ tablespoons Dijon mustard 1½ tablespoons nectar 2 garlic cloves, minced ¾ cup Panko breadcrumbs 2 tablespoons hacked new parsley 1 teaspoon lemon zing 1 tablespoon extra-virgin olive oil Four 6-ounce skinless salmon fillets Freshly ground dark pepper Sea salt, discretionary 2 tablespoons extra-virgin olive oil 6 cloves garlic minced 6 cups new infant spinach ½ teaspoon fit salt ¼ teaspoon newly ground dark pepper Lemon cuts for embellish.

Instructions:

1 Preheat the oven at 400 degrees F. Shower a gigantic planning dish with nonstick olive oil cooking sprinkle.

2 In a little bowl, whisk together the Dijon mustard, nectar, and garlic. In the second bowl, mix the breadcrumbs, parsley, and lemon punch. By then, shower in the olive oil to the bread piece mix and mix. Brush the most elevated mark of each salmon filet with the nectar mix, and a while later, dunk in the bread piece mix to cover. Put salmon fillets in an alone layer on a getting ready dish in the oven and cook for around 15 minutes until the salmon is cooked through.

3 While the salmon is warming, set up the spinach. Warmth oil over medium-high warmth in a fried dish. Add the garlic and cook for 1 min.

4 Add spinach, natural salt, and dim pepper. Toss the spinach for 1 to 2 minutes until by and large wilted.

5 Remove from warmth and present with salmon with lemon wedges as a bit of hindsight.

Serving per person: Calories 500; Total fat: 28g; Saturated fat: 7 g; Cholesterol: 85 mg; Sodium: 370 mg; Carbohydrates: 22g; Fiber: 2g; Sugar: 6g; Protein: 37g

TIP: Salmon is an essential fish to design, tastes uncommon, and is unnecessarily nutritious. Salmon is low in mercury and stacked with good omega-3 fat. Buy wild overdeveloped, if open.

Farro Salad

PREP TIME: 10 MIN

COOK TIME: 20 MIN

YIELD: 4 SERVINGS

INGREDIENTS

4 tablespoon extra-virgin olive oil, isolated 2 cups entire farro, flushed 6 cups water 4 cups natural child arugula 4 tablespoons new dill, cleaved 1 cup frozen peas, defrosted 4 ounces feta cheddar, disintegrated.

Dressing

3 tablespoons new lemon juice 1 teaspoon lemon zing

Bearings

1 Place 1 tablespoon of the olive oil in a medium pot over medium warmth. Permit olive oil to stew in the dish. Add the farro to stewing olive oil and mix until fragrant for around 3 minutes. 2 Add water and run of salt. Heat water to the point of boiling, cover, and lessen warmth to low. Permit to stew for around 35 minutes or until the farro is delicate and chewy (still somewhat firm). 3 Drain the farro is utilizing a fine-network strainer. Spread across a rimmed heating sheet to cool at room temperature. 4 Use an enormous serving bowl to make

a plate of mixed greens dressing. Whisk together the 3 leftover tablespoons of olive oil, 3 tablespoons of lemon juice, 1 teaspoon of lemon zing, ½ teaspoon of salt, and ¼ teaspoon of pepper. Put in a safe spot. 5 In an enormous serving bowl, add the arugula, farro, dill, and peas. Throw the fixings and sprinkle with feta and pour in the dressing.

PER SERVING: Calories 500; Total fat: 19g; Saturated fat: 5g; Cholesterol: 10mg; Sodium: 590mg; Carbohydrates: 69g; Fiber: 8g; Sugar: 3g; Protein: 20g.

TIP: Farro is a very nutritious old grain. Supermarkets typically sell three sorts of farro: pearled, semi-pearled, and entirety. Make sure to purchase the entire adaptation.

Cheesy Bean Burrito

PREP TIME: 15 MIN

COOK TIME: 5 MIN

YIELD: 1 SERVING

INGREDIENTS

2 teaspoons extra-virgin olive oil 1 clove garlic, slashed ½ little onion, cut slender 4 ounces (about ¼ of a can make dark beans, washed and depleted) ½ red ringer pepper, cleaved 2 tablespoons sweet corn portions, frozen 1 plum tomato, hacked into tiny pieces ¼ cup destroyed cheddar jack cheddar, diminished fat One 10-inch flour tortilla ¼ cup new salsa.

Preparations

1 In a large skillet, add the olive oil, garlic, onion, and sauté over medium-high warmth until the onion is transparent and daintily seared. Add the beans, red pepper, corn, tomato, and heat until the combination has warmed, and corn has thawed out (around 5 minutes), mixing sporadically.2 To make the burrito, take one large flour tortilla, add the bean mixture, and top with shredded cheese. Roll the tortilla and heat it in the microwave for 30 seconds until the cheese has melted. Top with salsa and serve.

PER SERVING: Calories 480; Total fat: 16g; Saturated fat: 4.5g; Cholesterol: 5mg; Sodium: 940mg; Carbohydrates: 72g; Fiber: 10g; Sugar: 11g; Protein: 17g.

TIP: Use a fruit salsa, such as mango, to add extra flavor and nutrients.

Whole Grain Linguini with Cannellini Beans

PREP TIME: 10 MIN

COOK TIME: 15 MIN

YIELD: 4 SERVINGS

INGREDIENTS

8 ounces entire grain linguini 2 tablespoons extra-virgin olive oil One 14.5-ounce can unimposing diced tomatoes One 15-ounce can cannellini beans, washed and depleted 3 tablespoons bumped pesto sauce 3 tablespoons escapades 1 tablespoon destroyed Parmesan cheddar.

DIRECTIONS

1. Cook the pasta according to rules; drain and set aside in a large pasta bowl. 2 In a large skillet, heat the olive oil over medium heat. Add the diced tomatoes and beans and simmer for about 5 minutes until heated. Stir in the pesto and heat for another few minutes. 3 Stir in the capers and remove from the heat. Add the sauce to the pasta, tossing gently to coat. Top with grated Parmesan if desired.

PER SERVING: Calories 470; Total fat: 25g; Saturated fat: 2.5g; Cholesterol: 0mg; Sodium: 900mg; Carbohydrates: 70g; Fiber: 7g; Sugar: 4g; Protein: 17g.

TIP: Rinse the beans several times with water to eliminate much of the excessive sodium typically added to canned beans.

Fudge Brownies

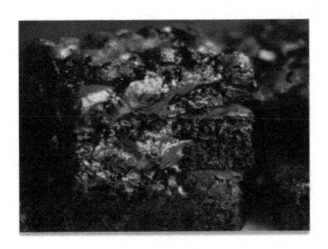

Ingredients

2 cups flour 2 cups sugar ½ cup of cocoa powder 1 teaspoon baking powder ½ teaspoon salt 1 cup vegetable oil 1 cup of water 1 teaspoon vanilla 1 cup dairy-free chocolate chips (optional) ½ cup chopped walnuts (optional)

Instructions

Preheat stove to 350°F and oil a 9 x 13-inch heating skillet. Add dry fixings in a blending bowl. Whisk together wet fixings and overlap into the dry fixings. Whenever wanted, including a large portion of the chocolate chips and cleaved pecans along with everything else. Empty blend into the readied container and sprinkle with outstanding chocolate chips and pecans, if utilizing. For fudge-like brownies, prepare for 20-25 minutes. For cake-like brownies, heat 25-30 minutes. Allow the brownies to cool somewhat before serving.

Nutritional Facts

Servings per container 9 Prep Total 10 min Serving Size 2/3 cup (70g) Amount per serving Calories 10 % Daily Value Total Fat 20g 2% Saturated Fat 2g 10% Trans Fat 4g - Cholesterol 10% Sodium 50mg 12%Total Carbohydrate 7g 20% Dietary Fiber 4g 7% Total Sugar 12g - Protein 3g Vitamin C 2mcg 19% Calcium 260mg 20% Iron 8mg 8% Potassium 235mg 6%

POMEGRANATE QUINOA PORRIDGE

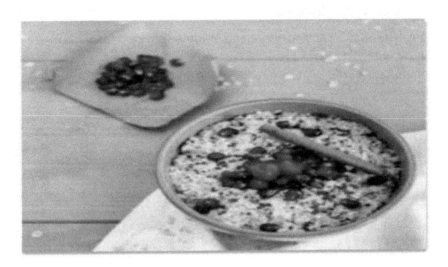

Ingredients

1/2 cup quinoa drops 2 1/2 teaspoons cinnamon 1 teaspoon vanilla concentrate 10 natural prunes, hollowed and cut into 1/4's 1 pomegranate mash 1/4 cup dried up coconut Stewed apples Coconut chips to embellish.

Instructions:

Gently place quinoa & almond milk into a saucepan & stir on medium to low heat for 9 minutes, until it smooth Add cinnamon, desiccated coconut & vanilla extract & taste Pit prunes & cut into quarters, add to porridge, and stir in well. Serve in individual bowls. Add a scoop of stewed apples (kindly view recipe below), pomegranates, prunes & coconut flakes. Ready to eat!

Stewed apples

Peel, core, slice apples, and place into a saucepan with water. Cook apples on medium heat until incredibly soft Remove from heat, drain & mash apples. Ready to serve and enjoy your breakfast!

Sweet Corn Soup

Ingredients

6 ears of corn 1 tablespoon corn oil 1 small onion 1/2 cup grated celery root 7 cups water or vegetable stock Add salt to taste.

Instructions:

Shuck the corn & slice off the kernels. In a large soup pot, put in the oil, onion, celery root, and one water cup. Let that mixture stew under low heat until the onion is soft. Add the corn, salt & remaining water and bring it to a boil. Cool briefly & then puree in a blender, then wait for it to cool before putting it through a food mill. Reheat & add salt with pepper to taste nice.

MEXICAN AVOCADO SALAD

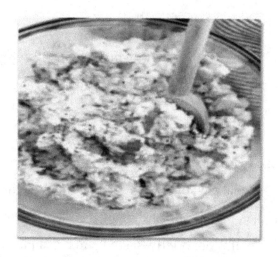

Ingredients

24 cherry tomatoes quartered 2 tablespoons extra-virgin olive oil 4 teaspoons red wine vinegar 2 teaspoons salt ¼ teaspoon freshly ground black pepper Gently chopped ½ medium yellow or white onion 1 jalapeño, seeded & finely chopped ¼ medium head iceberg lettuce, cut into ½-inch ribbons Chopped 2 ripe Hass avocados, seeded, peeled 2 tablespoons chopped fresh cilantro.

Instructions:

Add tomatoes, oil, vinegar, salt, & pepper in a neat medium bowl. Add onion, jalapeño & cilantro; toss well. Put lettuce on a platter & top with avocado Spoon tomato mixture on top and serve.

Crazy delicious raw pad thai

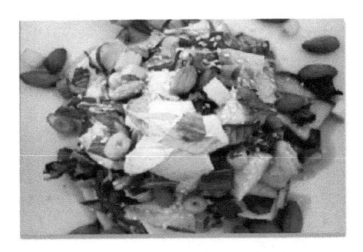

Ingredients

2 large zucchini Thinly sliced ¼ red cabbage Chopped ¼ cup fresh mint leaves Sliced 1 spring onion Peeled and sliced ½ avocado 10 raw almonds 4 tablespoons sesame seeds Dressing ¼ cup peanut butter 2 tablespoons tahini 2 lemons, juiced 2 tablespoons tamari / salt-reduced soy sauce, and add ½ chopped green chili

Instructions:

Collect dressing ingredients in a container, Pop the top on, and shake truly well to mix. I like mine pleasant and smooth. However, you can include a filtered water dash if it looks excessively thick. Using a mandolin or vegetable peeler, remove one external portion of skin from every zucchini and dispose of it. Combine zucchini strips, cabbage & dressing in a large mixing bowl, and blend well. Divide zucchini mix between two plates or bowls, Top with residual fixings, and enjoy it!

Kale and wild rice stir fly.

Ingredients

1 tablespoonful extra virgin olive oil Diced ¼ onion 3 carrots, cut into ½ inch slices 2 cups assorted mushrooms 2 bunch kale, chopped into bite-sized pieces 2 tablespoonful lemon juice 2 tablespoonful chili flakes, more if desired 1 tablespoon Braggs Liquid Aminos 2 cups wild rice, cooked.

Instructions:

In a large sauté pan, heat oil over on heater. Include onion & cook until translucent, for 35 to 10 minutes. Include carrots & sauté for another 2 minutes. Include mushrooms & cook for 4 minutes. Include kale, lemon juice, chili flakes & Braggs. Cook until kale is slightly wilted. Serve over wild rice and enjoy your Lunch!

Nutritional Facts

Servings per container 3 Prep Total 10 min Serving Size 2/3 cup (80g) Amount per serving Calories 220 % Daily Value Total Fat 5g 22% Saturated Fat 1g 8% Trans Fat 0g - Cholesterol 0% Sodium 200mg 7% Total Carbohydrate 12g 2%Dietary Fiber 1g 14% Total Sugar 12g - Protein 3g Vitamin C 2mcg 10% Calcium 20mg 1% Iron 2mg 2% Potassium 235mg 6%

Carpaccio

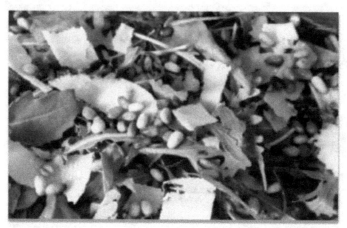

Nutrition Facts

Calories: 350 kcal | Gross carbohydrates: 3 g | Protein: 31 g | Fat: 24 g | Fiber: 1 g | Net carbohydrates: 2 g | Macro fat: 42 % | Macro proteins: 54 % | Macro carbohydrates: 4 % Total time: 5 minutes

Ingredients

100 grams of smoked prime rib 30 grams of arugula 20 grams of Parmesan cheese 10 grams of pine nuts 7 grams of butter 3 tablespoons olive oil with orange 1 tablespoon lemon juice pepper and salt

Instructions

Arrange the meat slices on a plate. Wash the arugula and pat dry or use a salad spinner. Place the arugula on top of the meat. Scrape some curls from the Parmesan cheese and spread them over the arugula. Put the butter in a small frying pan. Add the pine nuts as soon as the butter has melted. Let the pine nuts cook for a few minutes over medium heat, and then sprinkle them over the carpaccio. Make the vinaigrette by mixing the lemon juice into the olive oil—season with pepper and salt and drizzle over the carpaccio.

Keto spring frittata

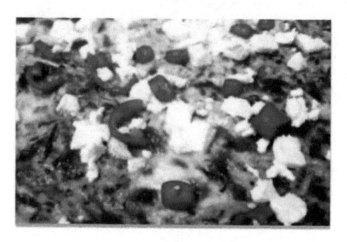

Total time: 15 minutes

Nutrition Facts

Calories: 955 kcal | Gross carbohydrates: 16 g | Protein: 46 g | Fats: 78 g | Fiber: 2 g | Net carbohydrates: 14 g | Macro fats: 57 % | Macro proteins: 33 % | Macro carbohydrates: 10 %

Ingredients

1 zucchini 0.5 bunch of mint 6 eggs Pinch of cayenne pepper 1 sprig of thyme or 1 teaspoon of dried thyme 80 grams of Pecorino cheese 0.5 red chili pepper 100 grams of feta cheese3 tablespoons extra virgin olive oil 0.25 teaspoon truffle oil optional Salt to taste

Salad

50 grams of watercress 0.5 stalks of celery 75 grams of fresh (raw) peas still in the pod 1 tablespoon lemon juice 2 tablespoons extra virgin olive oil 200 grams of herb cheese or Boursin

Instructions

Frittata: If you have a broiler with a barbecue, turn the flame broil on at the most elevated setting. Mesh the zucchini by hand or in the food processor and put it in a bowl. Sprinkle some salt over the ground zucchini. Put the zucchini in a sifter and press the zucchini solidly so a portion of the dampness goes out. Wash the mint and wipe it off. Eliminate the leaves from the twigs and cut them into pieces. Add to the zucchini and combine as one. Warmth the olive oil in a little (skillet) over medium-high warmth. Add the zucchini when the oil is hot and spread over the dish. Lower the heat to direct. Spread the zucchini over the plate. Beat the eggs in the bowl and add the truffle oil, cayenne pepper, and thyme leaves. Mesh the pecorino and add half of the pecorino to the bowl—beat eggs with thyme and cayenne pepper and truffle oil. Pour the beaten eggs over the zucchini in the skillet. Blend in the zucchini.

Decrease the warmth and stew for 5 minutes while making the plate of mixed greens. Put the frittata in a preparing dish or sprinkle the pecorino's remainder over it on an enormous scale. Spot as high as conceivable in the stove, just beneath the barbecue, and earthy colored for 5 minutes. If you don't have a flame broil, let the frittata cook in the oven for 5 minutes with a top on the container. If you need the cheddar to dissolve, you can tenderly turn the frittata by putting a cover or plate on the skillet and afterward turning it over. Put frittata under the barbecue. Wash the stew pepper and eliminate the seeds. Cut into little rings and sprinkle over the frittata when it emerges from the stove.

Additionally, disintegrate the feta over the frittata. Serving of mixed greens Bring a pot of water to the bubble and add a spot of salt. Wash the watercress and wipe off.

Put it in a plate of mixed greens bowl. Wash the celery and cut it into 5 cm pieces and cut them into thin sticks (additionally utilize the celery leaves). Eliminate the peas from the cover and whiten them for 1-2 minutes in the bubbling water in the pot (the equivalent applies to frozen peas or snow peas). At that point, let them channel in a colander. If you have new peas from the pod, this isn't required. While the peas chill off, make a vinaigrette by blending lemon squeeze with additional virgin olive oil. Add the peas to the plate of mixed greens and pour the vinaigrette over it. Combine everything as one healthy.

Super-fast keto sandwiches

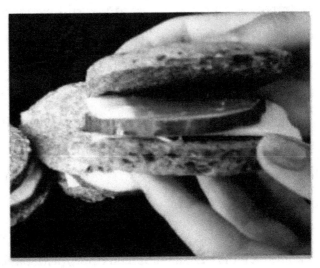

Nutrition Facts

Calories: 112 kcal | Gross carbohydrates: 2 g | Protein: 9 g | Fats: 6 g | Fiber: 5 g | Net carbohydrates: -3 g | Macro fat: 50 % | Macro proteins: 75 % | Macro carbohydrates: -25 % Total time: 10 minutes

Ingredients

1 teaspoon hemp flour 1 teaspoon almond flour 1 teaspoon of psyllium 1 teaspoon baking powder 1 egg at room temperature 1 teaspoon extra virgin olive oil or melted butter

Instructions

Put the dry ingredients in a cup and mix well. In particular, ensure that the baking powder is no longer visible. It helps if you put the baking powder through a (tea) strainer. Now add the egg and the butter. The egg must be at room temperature. If it is not, place it for about 10 minutes in a bowl with hot tap water. When you take the cup out, you want the top of the batter to be dry. If it is still wet, then put it in the microwave for a little longer. (If you place several cups in the microwave simultaneously, you may have to extend the time slightly depending on your type of microwave). Once the top is dry, remove the cup from the microwave and turn it on a cutting board. Decide now if you want thick rolls or something thinner. So, cut into 2 or 3 or 4 slices. Keep in mind that these slices must fit in your toaster. Now toast the bread slices in your toaster until they are firm but not hard. Your bread is now ready. You can use it immediately or use it for your breakfast or lunch the next day. Spread it well with butter so that you get enough fats.

Keto Croque Monsieur

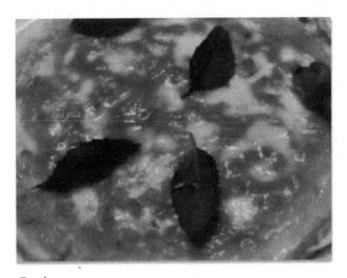

Total time: 7 minutes

Ingredients

2 eggs 25 grams of grated cheese 25 grams of ham 1 large slice 40 ml of cream 40 ml mascarpone 30 grams of butter Pepper and salt Basil leaves optional, to garnish.

Instructions

Beat the eggs in a bowl, add some salt and pepper. Add the cream, mascarpone, and grated cheese and stir together. Melt the butter over medium heat. The butter must not turn brown once the butter has melted, set the heat to low. Add half of the omelet mixture to the frying pan and immediately place the ham's slice on it. Now pour the rest of the omelet mixture over the ham and immediately put a lid on it. Allow 2-3 minutes of fry over low heat until the top is slightly firmer. Slide the omelet onto the cover to turn the omelet. Then put the omelet back in the frying pan to fry for another 1-2 minutes on the other side (still on low heat), then put the lid back on the pan. Don't let the omelet cook for too long! It does not matter if it is still liquid. Garnish with a few basil leaves if necessary.

Keto wraps with cream cheese and salmon

Nutrition Facts

Calories: 479 kcal | Gross carbohydrates: 4 g | Protein: 16 g | Fats: 45 g | Net carbohydrates: 4 g | Macro fats: 69 % | Macro proteins: 25 % | Macro carbohydrates: 6 % Total time: 10 minutes

Ingredients

80 grams of cream cheese 1 tablespoon dill or other fresh herbs 30 grams of smoked salmon 1 egg 15 grams of butter Pinch of cayenne pepper Pepper and salt

Instructions

Beat the egg well in a bowl. With 1 egg, you can make two flimsy encloses with a bit of skillet. Dissolve the spread over medium warmth in a bit of skillet. When the margarine has softened, add half of the beaten egg to the container. Move the skillet to and fro, so the whole base is covered with a skinny egg layer. Turn down the warmth! Cautiously extricate the egg on the edges with a silicone spatula and turn the thin omelet when the egg is done dribbling (around 45 seconds to 1 moment). You can do this by sliding it onto a top or plate and afterward sliding it back into the dish. Leave the opposite side alone cooked in around 30 seconds and later eliminated from the container. The omelet should be pretty light yellow. Rehash for the remainder of the beaten egg. When the omelets are prepared, they can cool on a cutting board or plate and make the filling. Cut the dill into tiny pieces and put it in a bowl. Add the cream cheddar and the salmon, cut them into small pieces. Combine as one. Add a smidgen of cayenne pepper and blend well. Taste briefly and afterward seasons with salt and pepper. Spread a layer on the wrap and move it up. Cut the wrap down the middle and keep it in the cooler until you eat it.

Savory keto broccoli cheese muffins

Nutrition Facts

Calories: 349 kcal | Gross carbohydrates: 4 g | Protein: 28 g | Fats: 25 g | Fiber: 1 g | Net carbohydrates: 3 g | Macro fat: 45 % | Macro proteins: 50 % | Macro carbohydrates: 5 % Preparation time: 10 minutes

Ingredients

4 eggs 75 grams of Parmesan cheese 125 grams of fresh cheese 125 grams of mozzarella 75 grams of broccoli 1.5 teaspoon baking powder 0.25 teaspoon garlic powder 0.25 teaspoon mustard

Instructions

Preheat the broiler to 160 ° Celsius. Cut the broccoli into tiny pieces. Carry a pot with water to the bubble, and when the water bubbles, add the broccoli pieces to the skillet. Whiten the broccoli for 1 moment in the bubbling water. Channel the broccoli well in a colander. Mesh the Parmesan cheddar and the new cheddar. Cut the mozzarella into tiny pieces. Beat the eggs well in a bowl. Add the cheddar, broccoli, and mustard to the eggs. Combine well as one. At that point, add the garlic powder and preparing powder and mix well once more. Add garlic powder and preparing powder. Preferably fill a silicone biscuit plate with the broccoli-cheddar egg player and heat for 10 minutes. You can likewise utilize paper biscuit cases. However, they are hard to eliminate. Prepare the biscuits in the preheated broiler until done. On the off chance that you put a stick in a biscuit, it should tell the truth (without hitter). At that point, your biscuits are prepared. Check if the biscuit is cooked with a satay stick.

Rusk

Nutrition Facts

Calories: 53 kcal | Gross carbohydrates: 1 g | Protein: 2 g | Fats: 4 g | Fiber: 0 g | Net carbohydrates: 1 g | Macro fats: 57 % | Macro proteins: 29 % | Macro carbohydrates: 14 % Time: 9 minutes

Ingredients

35 grams of almond flour 1 egg 1 tablespoon butter 0.5 teaspoon baking powder 1/8 teaspoon of salt

Instructions

Preheat the oven to 200° Celsius. Put all the ingredients in a cup and mix them well together with a fork. You want a narrower, higher cup that can go into the microwave. Put the cap on the most elevated position of the microwave for 90 seconds. Allow the dough to cool for a few minutes, and then place it on a cutting board. Cut the dough into 5 equal slices and place them on a baking sheet on a baking sheet. Bake for 5-6 minutes until golden and crispy.

Flaxseed hemp flour bun

Total time: 8 minutes

Nutrition Facts

Calories: 182kcal | Gross carbohydrates: 5 g | Protein: 11g | Fats: 15g
Fiber: 12 g | Net carbohydrates: -7g | Macro fats: 79% | Macro
proteins: 58% | Macro carbohydrates: -37%

Ingredients

1 teaspoon hemp flour 1 teaspoon linseed flour 1 teaspoon of psyllium
1 teaspoon baking powder 1 egg at room temperature 0.5 teaspoon
butter or mild olive oil or ghee

Instructions

Preheat the oven to 180 ° C (hot air oven) if you want to bake in the
oven, otherwise use a toaster. Put all dry ingredients in a large cup or
bowl that can be put in the microwave. Mix everything together.
Ensure that you no longer see the baking powder (so no white lumps),
or put the baking powder through a sieve. Add the egg and the butter
(melted but not necessary) and mix well. Put in the microwave on the
highest setting for 1 minute. The dark bun in the photo is this bun.
Remove the sandwich from the cup and halve or cut it into three slices.
Bake those slices for 5 minutes in the preheated oven or bake them in
a toaster.

muffins with Roquefort

Nutrition Facts

Calories: 160kcal | Gross carbohydrates: 2g | Protein: 6g | Fats: 14g
Fiber: 1g | Net carbohydrates: 1 g | Macro fats: 67% | Macro proteins:
29% | Macro carbohydrates: 5% Total time: 18 minutes

Ingredients

150 grams of zucchini 50 ml extra virgin olive oil Pepper to taste 100
grams of red pepper 75 grams of Roquefort 100 grams of mascarpone
6 eggs 1.5 teaspoons baking powder.

Instructions

Preheat the stove to 175 ° Celsius. Wash the zucchini and ringer
pepper and wipe off. Eliminate the seeds from the ringer pepper and
cut the chime pepper and zucchini into tiny shapes. Warmth the olive
oil in a skillet over medium-high heat and fry the zucchini and ringer
pepper in around 5 minutes to mollify. Beat the eggs with the heating
powder. You don't need any chunks of heating powder, so you should
either beat quite well or prepare powder through a tea sifter first.
Blend the vegetables, the player, mascarpone, and cheddar together
and afterward partition over the biscuit tins. Prepare for 15 minutes in
the preheated broiler. Check with a satay stick if they are finished. On
the off chance that you put the post in a biscuit, it should come out
dry. You need to allow the biscuits to prepare somewhat more on the
off chance that you actually have the hitter.

Wrap

Nutrition Facts

Calories: 128 kcal | Gross carbohydrates: 1 g | Protein: 6g | Fats: 12g
Fiber: 0.3 g | Net carbohydrates: 1 g | Macro fats: 64% | Macro
proteins: 32% | Macro carbohydrates: 4% Total time: 5 minutes

Ingredients

1 egg 0.5 teaspoons coconut oil or mild olive oil or butter 0.5 teaspoon
curry powder or other herbs or spices

Instructions

Warmth the coconut fat (or gentle olive oil or margarine) in a bit of
skillet over high warmth. Put the egg in a bowl and add the curry
powder and some salt. Beat it well with a fork or whisk. Turn down
the heat now. Empty the hitter into the skillet and slant the container
a little, so the player runs out and covers the whole lower part of the
dish. Prepare this thin omelet in 10-20 seconds. Cautiously eliminate
(with a scoop) the edges of the wrap from the sides of the skillet. Turn
the fold around and heat for a couple of moments on the opposite side.
When the edges begin to twist up, eliminate it from the container (this
is quick!).

Notes

If you make several wraps, you only have to put some oil in the pan
the first time.

Chapter 3: Dinner Recipes

Creamy Avocado Pasta

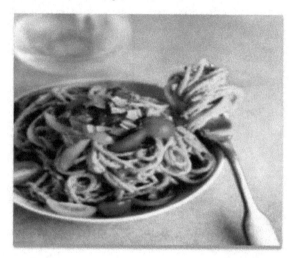

Ingredients

340 g / 12 oz. spaghetti 2 ripe avocados, halved, seeded & neatly peeled 1/2 cup fresh basil leaves 3 cloves garlic 1/3 cup olive oil 2-3 Teaspoons freshly squeezed lemon juice Add sea salt & black pepper, to taste 1.5 cups cherry tomatoes, halved.

Directions:

1. In an enormous pot of bubbling salted water, cook pasta as indicated by the bundle. At the point when still somewhat firm, channel and put in a safe spot.

2. To make the avocado sauce, consolidate avocados, basil, garlic, oil, and lemon juice in the food processor. Mix on high until smooth season with salt and pepper to taste.

3. In an enormous bowl, join pasta, avocado sauce, and cherry tomatoes until equally covered.

4. To serve, top with extra cherry tomatoes, new basil, or lemon zing.

5. Best when new. Avocado will oxidize after some time, so store extras in a concealed holder in more relaxed for one day.

Nutritional Facts

Servings per container 7 Prep Total 10 min Serving Size 2/3 cup (25g) Amount per serving Calories 19 % Daily Value Total Fat 8g 300% Saturated Fat 1g 40% Trans Fat 0g 20% Cholesterol 6%Sodium 210mg 3% Total Carbohydrate 22g 400% Dietary Fiber 4g 1% Total Sugar 12g 02.20% Protein 3g Vitamin C 2mcg 20% Calcium 10mg 6% Iron 4mg 7% Potassium 25mg 6%

BLACK BEAN VEGAN WRAPS

Ingredients

1 1/2 half cups of beans (sprouted & cooked) 2 carrots 1 or 2 tomatoes 2 avocadoes 1 cob of corn 1 Kale 2 or 3 sticks of celery 2 persimmons 1 Coriander Dressing: 1 Hachiya Persimmon (or half a mango) Juice of 1 lemon 2 to 3 tablespoons original olive oil 1/4 clean cup water 1 or 2 teaspoons grated fresh ginger 1/2 teaspoon of salt

Instructions:

Sprout & cook the black beans. Chop all the ingredients & mix them in a neat bow with the black beans. Mix all the ingredients for the dressing & pour them into the salad. Serve a spoonful in a clean lettuce leaf that you can easily roll into a wrap. Most people use iceberg or romaine lettuce.

ZUCCHINI PASTA WITH PESTO SAUCE

Ingredients

1 to 2 medium zucchinis (make noodles with a mandoline or spiralizer) 1/2 teaspoon of salt

For Pesto

Soaked 1/4 cup cashews Soaked 1/4 cup pine nuts 1/2 cup spinach 1/2 cup peas you can make it fresh or frozen one 1/4 cup broccoli 1/4 cup basil leaves 1/2 avocado 1 or 2 tablespoons original olive oil 2 tablespoons nutritional yeast 1/2 teaspoon salt Pinch black pepper.

Instructions:

Spot zucchini noodles in a sifter over a perfect bowl. Include 1/2 teaspoon of salt and sit while setting up the pesto sauce. Mix every one of the pesto sauce elements, Extract overabundance water from zucchini noodles and spot them in a perfect bowl. Pour the sauce on top and embellishment with some basil leaves and pine nuts.

BALSAMIC BBQ SEITAN AND TEMPEH RIBS

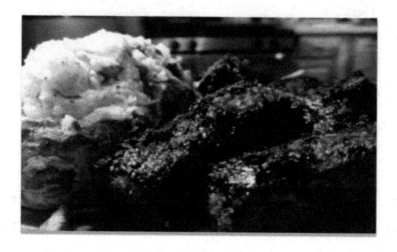

Ingredients

For the spice rub

1/4 cup raw turbinado sugar 1 or 2 tablespoons this should be smoked paprika 1 tablespoon cayenne pepper Minced 3 garlic cloves 2 tablespoons dried oregano 2 tablespoons Kosher salt 2 ½ tablespoons ground black pepper Minced ¼ cup fresh parsley.

Instructions

In a perfect bowl, blend the elements for the flavor rub. Mix well and set to the side. In a bit of pot over medium warmth, consolidate the squeezed apple vinegar, balsamic vinegar, maple syrup, ketchup, red onion, garlic, and chile. Blend and let stew sit, uncovered, for around an hour. Increment the level of the warmth to medium-high and cook for 15 extra minutes until the sauce thickens. Blend it regularly. If it seems, by all accounts, to be exorbitantly thick, incorporate some water—Preheat the stove to 350 degrees. In a spotless bowl, blend the dry elements for the seitan and mix well. In a perfect bowl, add the wet fixings. Add the wet fixings to the dry and mix until just combined. Control the dough gently until everything is consolidated and the batter feels flexible. Oil or shower a getting ready dish. Incorporate the butter into the heating dish, smoothing it, and extending it to fit the container.

Slice the mixture into 7 to 9 strips, and, after that, down the center to make 16 thick ribs. Top the mix with the flavor rub and back focus on it a piece. Warmth the seitan for 40 minutes to an hour or until the seitan has a solid surface to it. Eliminate the dish from the radiator. Recut the strips and circumspectly eliminate them from the preparing dish. Increment the broiler temperature to around 400 degrees. Slather the ribs with BBQ sauce and lay them on a preparing sheet. Set the ribs back in the warmer for approximately 12 minutes so the sauce can get somewhat cooked. Of course, you can cook the sauce-covered ribs on a barbecue or in a flame broil skillet.

GREEN BEAN CASSEROLE

Ingredients

Diced 1 large onion 3 tablespoons of original olive oil ¼ cup flour 2 cups of water 1 tablespoons of salt ½ tablespoons of garlic powder 1 or 2 bags frozen green beans (10 ounces each) 1 fried onion.

Instructions:

Preheat the broiler to 350 degrees. Warmth unique olive oil in a shallow container. Incorporate onion and mix at times while the onions mellow and turn transparent. This takes around 15 to 20 minutes, don't surge it since it gives such a lot of flavor! When the onion is all around cooked, incorporate the flour and mix well to cook the flour. It will be a dry blend. Incorporate salt and garlic powder. Add some water. Let stew for around 1 – 2 minutes and permit the combination to thicken. Promptly eliminate from heat. Empty green beans into a square heating dish and add 2/3 containers of onions. Incorporate the entirety of the sauce and mix well together. Spot in the stove and cook for 25 to 30 minutes. The sauce blend will be effervescent. Top with staying seared onions and cook for 4 to 12 minutes more. Serve promptly and make the most of your supper.

SOCCA PIZZA [VEGAN]

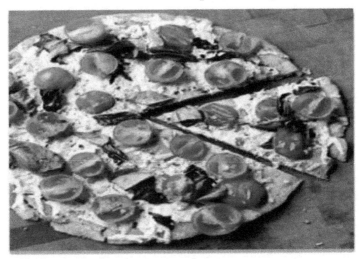

Ingredients

Socca Base 1 cup chickpea (garbanzo bean) flour – I used bob's Red Mill Garbanzo Fava Flour 1 or 2 cups of cold, filtered water 1 to 2 tablespoons of minced garlic ½ tablespoon of sea salt 2 tablespoons of coconut oil (for greasing) Toppings Add Tomato-paste Add Dried Italian herbs (oregano, basil, thyme, rosemary, etc.) Add Mushrooms Add Red Onion Add Capsicum/bell pepper Add Sun-dried tomatoes Add Kalamata olives Add Vegan Cheese & Chopped Fresh basil leaves.

Instructions:

Pre-heat oven to 350F. In a clean mixing bowl, whisk together garbanzo bean flour & water until no lumps are remaining. Stir together in garlic and sea salt. Allow resting for about 12 minutes to thicken. Grease 2 - 4 small, shallow dishes/tins with original coconut oil. Pour mixture into a clean dish & bake for about 20 - 15 minutes or until golden brown. Remove plates from the oven, top with your favorite toppings & vegan cheese (optional) & return to the oven for another 7 - 10 minutes or so. Remove dishes from the oven & allow to sit for about 2 – 5 minutes before removing pizzas from the containers. Enjoy your dinner!

Mediterranean salad with quinoa and rocket

Nutrition Facts

Time: 20 min kcal: 401 KH: 23 g E: 6 g Q: 30 g

Ingredients

40 grams of quinoa 1 lime freshly pressed 60 g paprika, green, fresh 60 g small cucumber 1 tomato / n 1 small onion, red50 g olives black raw 50g rocket, new 2 stems of basil fresh 1 small parsnip raw 4 tablespoons olive oil 1 pinch of sea salt (Fleur de sell) 1 pinch of pepper, black.

Preparation

Put the quinoa in a strainer and wash with running water to eliminate any harsh substances. Cover the quinoa in a pan with water and stew for 8 - 10 minutes. At that point, channel and leave the granules in the container. Season the quinoa with a lime squeeze, salt, and pepper. Eliminate paprika from portions and dividers and cut them into tiny pieces. Peel the cucumber and cut it into small pieces. Cut tomato into little pieces. Peel the onion and cut it into thin rings. Strip and cut the parsnip. Wash the rucola leaves and channel well, eliminate them for a really long-time closes Wash the basil and shake dry; at that point, strip off the plates. Blend the quinoa, paprika, cucumber, tomato, onion, parsnip, rocket, and olives in a bowl. Add the olive oil and season with salt and pepper. Put the serving of mixed greens on two plates and sprinkle with basil leaves.

Baked chicken thighs in lemon sage butter

Nutrition Facts

Time: 50 min kcal: 793 KH: 5 g E: 48g F: 63 g

Ingredients

3 chicken thighs, with skin and bones 2 lemon/n 10 stems of thyme new 2 stalks of rosemary new 2 stems of sage fresh100 g of margarine 2 tbsp. olive oil 1 teaspoon ocean salt (Fleur de sel) 1 touch of pepper, dark 10 garlic toes

Readiness

Separate chicken thighs, for example, release the thighs from the lower leg Season with salt and pepper Wash the spices and shake dry Crush the garlic cloves unpeeled with the level side of the blade. Wash and cut the lemons. Heat the olive oil in the skillet and add the meat with spices, lemons, and garlic. Fry the meat in general, at that point, place in the search for gold minutes at 175 ° C in the preheated stove. At that point, eliminate the skillet from the broiler and take out the bits of meat. Put the margarine in the skillet and heat to the end of boiling. Set the beef back into the dish and sprinkle the spread with the spoon a few times over the heart.

Zucchini pasta with pesto

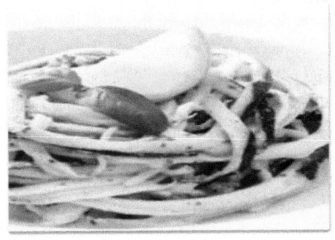

Nutrition Facts

2Time: 20 min kcal: 449 KH: 12 g E: 16g F: 35 g

Ingredients

500 g of zucchini 50 g paprika, yellow, fresh 30 g of cashew nuts 40 g Ricotta Magerstufe 30 g of Parmesan 1 tsp. turmeric, powder1 pinch of sea salt (Fleur de sel) 1 pinch of pepper, black 50 g of olive oil

Preparation

Wash the peppers, eliminate the centers and parcels and cut into wide strips. Spot the paprika segments on a preparing sheet with the skin side up and broil under the barbecue for 8 - 10 minutes at 200 ° C until the skin tosses bubbles. At that point, eliminate the tin, cover the pepper strips with a sodden dishcloth and permit them to cool somewhat. Cautiously eliminate the skin. Broil the cashews in a skillet until brilliant earthy colored, in the middle panning a few times. Put the cashews, paprika, ricotta, coarsely ground Parmesan, turmeric, salt, pepper, and olive oil in a shaker and puree with the hand blender. Wash and dry the zucchini; at that point, remove the finishes and make long zucchini noodles with the winding shaper. Whiten the zucchini noodles in a pot of bubbling salted water for a couple of moments, at that point, channel off the water. Add the pesto to the noodles and blend. At long last, season with salt and pepper once more. Fill the zucchini noodles on two plates and sprinkle them with newly pressed lemon juice.

Roasted pork steak with vegetables

Nutrition Facts

Time: 20 min kcal: 714 KH: 12 g E: 58 g F: 48 g

Ingredients

250 g pork chop, boneless 100 g zucchini, raw 40 g paprika, red, fresh 40 g paprika, yellow, fresh 40 g paprika, green, fresh 50 g mushrooms, brown 5 stems of thyme, fresh 2 tbsp. Olive oil 1 tbsp. butter 1 pinch of sea salt (Fleur de sel) 1 pinch of pepper, black

Preparation

Wash vegetables and drain Slice zucchini at an angle Cut peppers into strips Clean and halve mushrooms Wash the thyme and shake dry. Put the pork chop in the hot grill pan, add the thyme, and grill the meat from both sides. Heat butter and oil in the second pan and fry the zucchini, peppers, and mushrooms. Season the vegetables with salt and pepper and place them on a plate Season the pork chop and add to the vegetables.

Salmon in cream sauce with peas and lemon

Nutrition Facts

Time: 25 min kcal: 1024 KH: 19 g E: 61 g Q: 78 g

Ingredients

500 g salmon filet, without skin 150 g peas green raw 200 ml whipped cream 30% 2 small shallots / n 1 toe garlic 20 g of Parmesan40 g of butter 1 lemon / n medium 1 pinch of nutmeg 1 pinch of pepper, white 1 pinch of sea salt

Preparation

Wash the salmon and pat dry, then cut them into bite-sized pieces. Peel the shallots and finely dice. Peel the garlic and finely chop. Heat the butter in the pan, add shallots and garlic and fry the salmon pieces in it. Add the cream and stir. Add the peas and simmer briefly over medium heat.

Meanwhile, wash the lemon hot, dry, and rub the bowl with the grater. Halve the lemon and squeeze out the juice. Add grated Parmesan, lemon peel, and a little nutmeg to the pan and stir. Season with lemon juice, salt, and pepper.

Steamed vegetable pan

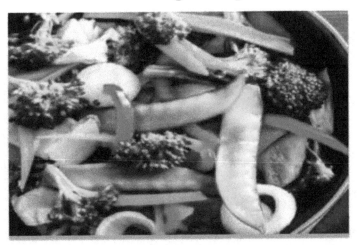

Nutrition Facts

Time: 10 min kcal: 239 KH: 27 g E: 9 g F: 10g

Ingredients

100 g of broccoli 50 g paprika, red, fresh 50 g paprika, yellow, fresh 50 g onion 100 g Kaiserschoten, fresh 2 medium carrots 1 pinch of sea salt (Fleur de sel) 1 tbsp. olive oil

Preparation

Wash the broccoli and cut the florets from the stalk. Remove the peppers from the seeds and partitions and cut them into strips. Peel the onion and cut it into rings. Wash and drain the pears. Peel the carrot and cut it into thin sticks. Heat the olive oil in the pan. Put the prepared vegetables in the pan and fry them all over, stirring several times. Season everything with salt and serve.

Chicken breast with pan vegetables

Nutrition Facts

Time: 30 min kcal: 382 KH: 17 g E: 48g Q: 11 g

Ingredients

180 g chicken breast, without skin 80 g Brussels sprouts 120 g carrot 120 g onion 1 pinch of sea salt (Fleur de sel) 1 pinch of pepper, black 1 tbsp. olive oil 1 stalk of parsley, fresh

Preparation

Wash chicken breast and pat dry Remove the dry stem and withered leaves from the sprouts, then halve each time. Peel carrot and slice. Peel the onion and cut it into pieces. Wash the parsley and shake dry, then chop. Heat the olive oil in the pan and fry the chicken breast from both sides until golden brown until the meat is cooked. Season the chicken breast with salt and pepper. Add the vegetables to the hot pan and fry, then season with salt and pepper. Place the chicken breast with the pan vegetables on a plate and sprinkle with Petersilia.

Frittata with spinach and grainy cream cheese

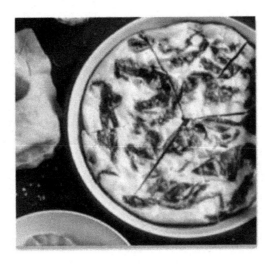

Nutrition Facts

Time: 40 min kcal: 399 KH: 3 g E: 28g Q: 30 g

Ingredients

4,00 eggs size M 30 g spinach, raw 3 tablespoons whipped cream 30% 50 g of Parmesan 100 g fine cream cheese, 20% fat i.Tr 1 pinch of sea salt (Fleur de sel)1 pinch of pepper, black 1 tbsp. olive oil

Preparation

Wash the spinach and drain well. Beat the eggs and stir in a bowl with whipped cream. Add the cream cheese and season with salt and pepper. Stir again. Heat the olive oil in the pan and add the egg mass. Add the spinach leaves and let the egg mass stagnate over medium heat. Then add freshly grated Parmesan cheese over the egg mass.

Place the frittata in the pan for 15 - 20 minutes in the oven preheated to 180 ° C. Remove the finished lemon juice and serve.

Mushroom pan with cream sauce and herbs

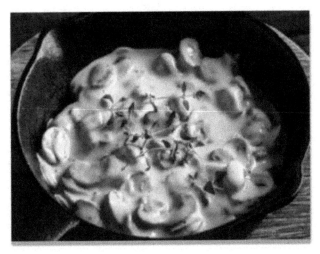

Nutrition Facts

Time: 15 min kcal: 431 KH: 11 g E: 10g Q: 39 g

Ingredients

250 g mushrooms, brown 100 g whipped cream 30% 10 g butter 2 toes of garlic 1 pinch of sea salt (Fleur de sel) 1 pinch of pepper, black1 pinch of nutmeg 1 shallot / n 1 stalk of oregano, fresh

Preparation

Brush the mushrooms, brush with a brush if necessary, and then cut off the stems' dry ends. Slice the mushrooms Peel the garlic and cut it into thin slices. Peel the shallot and dice finely. Heat the butter in the pan and sauté the shallot with garlic. Add mushrooms and fry everything for a few minutes. Add the cream and season everything with salt, pepper, and freshly grated nutmeg. Wash the oregano and shake it dry. Serve the mushroom frying pan with cream sauce and herbs.

False bulgur salad with paprika and fresh mint

Nutrition Facts

Time: 30 min kcal: 148 KH: 9 g E: 3 g F: 10g

Ingredients

300 g of cauliflower 80 g paprika, red, new 80 g paprika, yellow, fresh 80 g pepper, green, fresh 2 small tomatoes / n1 small onion, red 2 cloves of garlic 2 spring onions / n 5 stems of coriander, new 1 lemon / s freshly pressed 4 tablespoons olive oil 1 pinch of sea salt (Fleur de sel) 1 pinch of pepper, black 1 pinch cumin dried 2 stalks of mint.

Preparation

Wash the cauliflower, place in a pot with a steaming insert, and blanch for a few minutes; it should not be too soft. Grind cauliflower with the grater. Wash and drain the remaining vegetables and herbs. Cut the peppers into small cubes. Quarter the tomatoes, remove the stalk, and cut them into pieces. Peel the onion and cut it into thin rings. Cut the spring onions into rounds. Pick the leaves of coriander and mint from the stalk and chop them roughly. Place all prepared ingredients in a salad bowl. Add olive oil, a little lemon juice, cumin, salt, and pepper to the salad and mix. Season the salad and chill until it is consumed. For a better taste, the salad should have some time to sit.

Triple Decker Hummus Sandwich

PREP TIME: 10 MIN |

COOK TIME: 0 MIN

YIELD: 1 SERVING

INGREDIENTS

3 slices whole-grain or rye toast 1 tablespoon pesto 2 tablespoons hummus 1 cup baby arugula, organic 1 pitted avocado ½ teaspoon pepper 8 cherry tomatoes

DIRECTIONS

1 Toast three slices of whole grain or rye bread. 2 Mix pesto with hummus and then spread 1 tablespoon of pesto hummus onto each slice of bread. 3. Scoop out the avocado and portion. Sprinkle ½ teaspoon of pepper on top of the avocado for seasoning. 4 Slice the cherry tomatoes in flat halves. 5 Make your sandwich: layer bread, then hummus, then arugula, avocado, and tomato. Repeat then top with the last slice of bread, hummus side down. Cut in half for easier eating.

PER SERVING:

Calories 590; Total fat: 37g; Saturated fat: 7g; Cholesterol: 60mg; Sodium: 610mg; Carbohydrates: 61g; Fiber: 18g; Sugar: 6g; Protein: 17g.

TIP: Adding the arugula layer directly on top of the hummus and adding the avocado helps keep the ingredients in place. For extra flavor, add a squeeze of lemon juice on top of the hummus.

Whole Grain Linguini with Clams

PREP TIME: 10 MIN

COOK TIME: 20 MIN

YIELD: 4 SERVINGS

INGREDIENTS

12 ounces whole-grain linguini, uncooked 2 tablespoons extra-virgin olive oil 4 cloves garlic, sliced thinly ½ teaspoon crushed red pepper flakes ¼ cup dry white wine, preferably Sauvignon Blanc Two 6.5-ounce cans minced clams, drained (with liquid from cans reserved) ¼ cup fresh parsley, chopped 1 tablespoon fresh basil, chopped 4 tablespoons Parmesan cheese.

DIRECTIONS

1. Cook the linguini according to the instructions on the package until it's al dente, and then drain it well. Before emptying, put ½ cup pasta liquid aside. 2 In a large skillet, gently heat the oil over medium-low heat. Add the garlic and red pepper flakes and cook, constantly stirring until fragrant for about 15 to 20 seconds. 3. Add the reserved clam juice, white wine, and reserved pasta water to the skillet. Reduce the heat to low and simmer gently until the liquid begins to reduce, about 1 minute. 4 Add the clams and simmer until just heated for about 30 to 60 seconds. Then stir in the parsley and basil. 5 Add the pasta and

toss until it's well coated, about 30 to 45 seconds. Top with the grated Parmesan cheese and serve immediately.

PER SERVING: Calories 580; Total fat: 14 g; Saturated fat: 3 g; Cholesterol: 80 mg; Sodium: 240 mg; Carbohydrates: 68 g; Fiber: 1g; Sugar: 3 g; Protein: 50g

TIP: The salt used to preserve inexpensive cooking wine makes it unpotable. Better to use a real Sauvignon Blan

Bean and Turkey Slow Cooker Chili

PREP TIME: 10 MIN

COOK TIME: 4 HRS

YIELD: 4 SERVINGS

INGREDIENTS

1 tablespoon extra-virgin olive oil 1¼ pounds additional lean ground turkey bosom ½ medium onion, slashed Two 28-ounce can no-salt-added squashed tomatoes Two 16-ounce jars dim red kidney beans, flushed and depleted One 15-ounce can make dark beans, washed and depleted 2 tablespoons stew powder 1 teaspoon red pepper pieces ½ tablespoon garlic power ½ tablespoon ground cumin 1 squeeze ground dark pepper 1 squeeze ground allspice Salt to taste, discretionary.

Bearings

1. Heat the oil in a massive skillet over medium-high warmth. 2 Place the turkey and onions in the skillet and cook until equally sautéed around 5 minutes. 3 Coat within a sluggish cooker with a nonstick splash. 4 Mix together the turkey, squashed tomatoes, kidney beans, dark beans, and onion. Season with the bean stew powder, red pepper drops, garlic powder, cumin, dark pepper, and flavor and mix. 5 Cover and cook 4 hours on high. Serve hot. Add salt to taste.

PER SERVING: Calories 630; Total fat: 7g; Saturated fat: 1 g; Cholesterol: 70 mg; Sodium: 740 mg; Carbohydrates: 84g; Fiber: 12 g; Sugar: 15g; Protein: 60g

TIP: Serve warm, embellished with a bit of sans fat destroyed cheddar for flavor. On the off chance that you have the opportunity, cook the stew on low warmth for 8 hours. Stewing plans throughout longer timeframes separates each one of those discreet flavors.

Sweet Pomegranate Chicken with Couscous

PREP TIME: 10 MIN

COOK TIME: 15 MIN

YIELD: 4 SERVINGS

INGREDIENTS

extra-virgin olive oil 2 tablespoons 1 large red onion halved and thinly sliced 1 chicken bouillon cube Four 5-ounce chicken breasts 2 tablespoons harissa ¾ cup pomegranate juice ½ cup pomegranate seeds 1 cup couscous, preferably whole-wheat Dash ground black pepper Dash salt ½ cup toasted almond pieces ¼ cup mint, chopped.

DIRECTIONS

1 Heat the oil in a significant skillet on medium warmth. Add the red onions and mix. Disintegrate the chicken bouillon solid shape by hand and add to the cooking container with onions. Cook for a few minutes, permitting the onions to relax. 2 Push the onions aside from the box and add the chicken bosoms until they earthy colored on the sides. Flip the chicken and mix in the harissa and pomegranate juice. Let stew for 10 minutes, until the sauce thickens and chicken is cooked through. Mix in ¼ cup of pomegranate seeds. 3 To make the couscous, bubble 1¼ cups water in a pot or little pot. In an enormous bowl, add dry couscous with a touch of salt and pepper. Pour sufficient bubbling water to cover the couscous. Cover the bowl with a towel and put it in

a safe spot for 5 minutes. 4 After 5 minutes, cushion the couscous with a fork and mix in the almonds and mint. 5. Serve the chicken and sauce on top of the couscous combination and sprinkle the remaining ¼ cup pomegranate seeds on top.

PER SERVING: Calories 590; Total fat: 23g; Saturated fat: 2g; Cholesterol: 80mg; Sodium: 360mg; Carbohydrates: 54g; Fiber: 1g; Sugar: 15g; Protein: 45gTIP: To avoid excess sugar intake, be sure to use a pomegranate juice with no sugar added.

Chocolate Berry Protein Smoothie

PREP TIME: 5 MIN

COOK TIME: NONE

YIELD: 1 SERVING

INGREDIENTS

12 fluid ounces unsweetened vanilla almond milk 1 tablespoon peanut butter (can substitute with any nut/ seed butter) 1 tablespoon chia seeds ½ fresh banana ¼ cup frozen wild blueberries 1 scoop vegan chocolate protein powder.

DIRECTIONS

1 Place ingredients in a blender in the order listed. Blend until smooth and serve.

PER SERVING:

Calories 600; Total fat: 19g; Saturated fat: 2g; Cholesterol: 0 mg; Sodium: 780mg; Carbohydrates: 48g; Fiber: 8g; Sugar: 20g; Protein: 61g

TIP:

For extra nutrition and negligible extra calories, add in 3 ounces of frozen organic spinach.

Chapter 4: SNACKS RECIPES

Fried sea bream with fresh mango salsa

Nutritional Facts

Time: 30 min kcal: 326 KH: 15 g E: 37 g F: 13 g

Ingredients

4 small bream, fillet 100 g mango, raw 100 g cucumber with peel, raw100 g paprika, red, new 50 g spinach, basic 30 g of Parmesan, grated 1 pinch of sea salt (Fleur de sel) 1 pinch of pepper, black 1 g lemon / n 1 tbsp. olive oil.

Preparation

Wash bream and pat dry Peel the mango and cut the pulp into small slices. Wash the cucumber and cut it into small pieces. Remove the peppers from the seeds and partitions and cut them into small cubes. Wash the spinach and dry it in the salad spinner. Remove too long stalks from the spinach; wash and dry the lemon, then make lemon zest with the grater. Halve the lemon and squeeze out the juice. Mix mango, cucumber, paprika, and a little lemon juice in a bowl and season with salt and pepper. Put spinach leaves on two plates. Heat the olive oil in the frying pan and fry the bream fillets on both sides. Season the fillets with salt and pepper and sprinkle with freshly grated

Parmesan. Add the fish fillets to the spinach and serve together with the mango salsa.

Vital red cabbage salad with nuts and seeds

Nutritional Facts

Time: 10 min

kcal: 206 KH: 19 g E: 6 g F: 13 g Ingredients 150 g red cabbage, raw 20 g walnut kernels, fresh 1 tbsp. balsamic vinegar (balsamic vinegar) 1 teaspoon agave syrup, 1 pinch of sea salt (Fleur de sel), 1 pinch of pepper, black5 g of chard, raw

Preparation

For red cabbage, remove the outer leaves, then quarter with a knife, remove the stalk and cut it into great strips. Or a plane with the vegetable slicer in great strips. Add the balsamic, agave syrup, salt, and pepper to the bowl and mix. Rinse chard and dry. Put the red cabbage and chard in the bowl and mix with the dressing. Finely chop walnut kernels. Arrange red cabbage salad on a plate or in a bowl and serve with the chopped walnut kernels.

Omelet with eggplant and tomato

Nutritional Facts

Time: 20 min kcal: 416 KH: 8 g E: 29 g Q: 29 g

Ingredients

4 size M egg, from chicken, raw 100 g cherry tomatoes 50 g aubergine, natural 1 stalk of basil, fresh 1 tbsp whipped cream 30% 1 pinch of sea salt (Fleur de sel)1 pinch of pepper, black 1 tsp. olive oil

Preparation

Wash aubergine and tomatoes drain and slice. Lightly salt eggplant. Beat the eggs in a bowl and whisk with cream, a little salt, and pepper. Heat the oil in the pan and add the egg mass. Spread the aubergines and tomato slices on top. Put the lid on the pan and let everything fade. Season with salt and pepper and sprinkle with basil. Carefully fold the omelet in half and place it on a plate.

Chickpea salad with halloumi

Nutritional Facts

Time: 20 min kcal: 662 KH: 27 g E: 29 g F: 46 g

Ingredients

200 g of chickpeas 200 g Halloumi 1 shallot ½ spring onion / n 30 g of radish raw50 g tomato / n 50 g of cucumber 20 g of sweetcorn canned 4 stems of parsley 4 tablespoons olive oil 1 pinch of sea salt 1 pinch of pepper, black.

Preparation

Chickpeas in a colander and rinse under running water, then drain Heat pan and fry Halloumi from both sides until roast strips are recognizable Halloumi with salt and pepper remove from the pan and cut into pieces. Meanwhile, clean the radishes and cut them into thin slices. Wash tomatoes and cut them into pieces. Remove the peppers from the seeds and partitions and cut them into pieces. Wash the cucumber and cut it into small cubes. Peel the shallot and cut it into fine rings. Clean the spring onion and cut into rounds at an angle. Wash the parsley and shake it dry, then pluck the leaves and chop them. Remove the corn from the tin and drain. Put all the prepared salad ingredients in a bowl and mix. Add olive oil and some salt and pepper and stir again. Put the chickpeas salad with halloumi on two plates and serve.

Salad with chard, avocado, nuts, and feta

Nutritional Facts

Time: 10 min kcal: 447 KH: 10 g E: 14 g Q: 39 g

Ingredients

20 g of chard 60 g avocado, hate, fresh 50 g of tomatoes dried 30 g of feta 30 g walnut kernels, fresh 20 g onion, red 1 pinch of sea salt1 pinch of pepper, black.

Preparation

Wash the chard and drain well. Halve the avocado and remove the kernel, then peel the pulp and cut into small pieces. Cut the dried tomatoes into chunks. Crumble feta by hand. Chop walnuts. Peel onions and cut into rings. Put all the ingredients and the olive oil in a salad bowl and mix. Finally, season the salad with salt and pepper and place it on a plate.

Tuna with vegetables and avocado

Nutritional Facts

Time: 15 min kcal: 372 KH: 8 g E: 18 g Q: 29 g

Ingredients

1 can of tuna fillets natural, canned 1 avocado, hate, fresh 50 g paprika, red, new 50 g paprika, orange, fresh 50 g of cucumber 1 spring onion / n30 g of sweetcorn canned 6 stalks of parsley 50 g radishes raw ½ peppers (chili) essential 1 lime freshly pressed 2 tbsp. olive oil 1 pinch of nutmeg dried 1 pinch of sea salt (Fleur de sel) 1 bit of pepper, black.

Preparation

Open the tuna can a bit, drain the juice, and then open the tin entirely and cut the tuna into pieces with the fork. Halve the avocado and remove the kernel. Halve the lime and squeeze the juice. Sprinkle both avocado halves with a bit of lime juice. Peel the cucumber and cut it into pieces. Remove the peppers from the seeds and partitions and cut them into small cubes. Wash the tomatoes and cut them into pieces. Clean the spring onion and cut it into rings. Pour corn into a sieve and drain. Wash the parsley and shake it dry, then peel and chop the leaves. Chop the chili lengthwise and corer lengthwise, then chop finely. Clean the radish and cut it into small pieces. Put tuna, cucumber, peppers, tomatoes, spring onions, corn, parsley, radishes, and chili pepper in a bowl. Add olive oil and a little lime juice and season with freshly grated nutmeg, salt, and pepper. Mix the salad well, then serve together with the avocado.

Colorful vegetable salad

Nutritional Facts

Time: 30 min kcal: 239 KH: 10 g E: 4 g Q: 19g

Ingredients

200 g aubergine raw 150 g of tomato / n 40 g paprika, yellow, fresh 40 g paprika, red, new 25 g of endives salad 25 g Romanosalat1 small onion, red 1 small pepper (chili) raw 2 cloves of garlic 1 pinch of cumin 1 pinch of sea salt (Fleur de sel) 1 pinch of pepper, black 4 tablespoons olive oil

Preparation

Wash eggplant and dry, then cut into pieces. Peel garlic and squeeze with a garlic press. Mix aubergine with 1 tbsp. Olive oil, garlic, salt, and pepper in a bowl and spread on a baking sheet lined with baking paper. Eggplant for about 10 minutes at 160 ° Cook C in a preheated oven until soft.

Meanwhile, wash and quarter the tomatoes. Remove peppers from cores and partitions and cut into thin sticks. Wash lettuce leaves and shake dry, then cut into thin strips. Peel the onion and cut it into strips. Cut chili pepper into thin rings: mix tomatoes, peppers, lettuce, onion, and chili pepper in a salad bowl. Add the olive oil, cumin, salt, and pepper and mix well. Take the aubergine out of the oven, allow cooling briefly, and adding to the salad. Mix everything and place it on two plates.

Chickpea salad with tomatoes and cucumber

Nutritional Facts

Time: 10 min kcal: 153 KH: 10 g E: 4 g F: 10g

Ingredients

100 g of tomatoes 50 g of chickpeas 60 g of cucumber 10 g spring onion 1 tbsp olive oil Sea-salt pepper

Preparation

Wash tomatoes and cut them into pieces. Chickpeas in a colander and rinse under running water, then drain. Wash the cucumber and cut it into pieces. Clean spring onion and cut it into rings. Place tomatoes, chickpeas, cucumber, and spring onion in a salad bowl. Add olive oil and season with salt and pepper. Mix the salad and put it in a bowl.

Beefsteak with broccoli

Nutritional Facts

Time: 20 min kcal: 430 KH: 9 g E: 39g Q: 24 g

Ingredients

120 g beef fillet 60 g of broccoli 30 g pepper, red, fresh 2 cloves of garlic 1 onion, red 1 stalk of basil fresh1 stalk of rosemary 2 tbsp. olive oil 1 pinch of sea salt (Fleur de sel) 1 pinch of pepper, black

Preparation

Wash the peppers and cut them into strips. Peel the onion and cut it into rings. Peel and finely chop the garlic. Wash the herbs and shake dry, peel the leaves from the basil, and chop. Wash the broccoli and cut the florets from the stem. Add the broccoli to a pot of water and steam, bring the water to a boil and cook the vegetables with the lid closed for 5 to 8 minutes. Wash beef filet and dab dry. Heat the olive oil in the pan and add the filet with rosemary together. Fry the filet for 3 - 5 minutes, depending on the thickness and desired cooking point, then remove salt and pepper and briefly rest.

Meanwhile, add the pepper, onion, and garlic to the hot pan and sauté—season with salt and pepper. Arrange broccoli, pate, and beef fillet on a plate. Place the basil over the meat and serve.

Chicken thighs with vegetables

nutritional Facts

Time: 60 min kcal: 615 KH: 6 g E: 35g F: 48 g

Ingredients

4 chicken drumsticks, with skin and bones 100 g cherry tomatoes 100 g mushrooms, brown 1 onion 6 tbsp. olive oil 4 garlic toes 2 stalks of rosemary 1 teaspoon paprika, powder1 pinch of sea salt 1 pinch of pepper, black

Preparation

Wash the chicken drumsticks and wipe them off. Strip the onion and cut it into rings. Wash the rosemary and shake it dry. Pulverize the garlic cloves with the level side of the blade. Rub the chicken drumsticks done with olive oil, paprika, salt, and pepper. At that point, place the thighs along with onion and garlic in a flame-resistant form and spot the rosemary on them. Bubble thighs in a preheated broiler at 200 ° C for 30 minutes. At the same time, wash and divide the tomatoes. Clean and cut the mushrooms. Add both following 30 minutes to the thighs and cook everything for another 10 - 15 minutes until the thighs are cooked. At that point, serve the chicken drumsticks hot in the skillet.

Quinoa with roasted pumpkin

Nutritional Facts

Time: 30 min kcal: 266 KH: 32 g E: 7 g Q: 11 g

Ingredients

60g quinoa 200 g Hokkaido pumpkin ½ onion 50 g rocket 1 sprig of fresh mint Juice of half a lime 2 tbsp. olive oil pepper Sea-salt

Preparation

Spot the quinoa in a fine sifter and wash under running water to flush off the unpleasant substances. Cover the quinoa in a pan with water. Stew for 8 - 10 minutes until the granules are firm. Channel the quinoa and permit are dissipating. Wash and dry the pumpkin; at that point, cut down the middle and scratch out the seeds with a spoon. Cut the pumpkin into tiny pieces. Strip the onion, divide and cut it into thin rings. Wash the rocket and channel well. Warmth the oil in the skillet and sauté the pumpkin. Add the quinoa and onion and season with salt and pepper. Wash the mint and shake dry, strip off the leaves, and slash. Add the lime squeeze, rocket, and mint and combine everything as one.

Fresh Fruit

The health benefits of eating fresh fruit daily should not be minimized. So, make sure that you enjoy some in-season fruit as one of your daily vegan snacks.

Ingredients

: Chop your favorite fruit and make a fast and easy fruit salad, adding some squeezed orange juice to make a nice juicy dressing. Serve with some soy or coconut milk yogurt or vegan ice cream if desired. Top with some tasty walnuts or toasted slivered almonds to make it a sustaining snack.

Nutritional Facts

Servings per container 10 Prep Total 10 min Serving Size 5/5 Amount per serving Calories 1% % Daily Value Total Fat 24g 2% Saturated Fat 8g 3% Trans Fat 4g 2% Cholesterol 2% Sodium 10mg 22% Total Carbohydrate 7g 54%Dietary Fiber 4g 1% Total Sugar 1g 1% Protein 1g 24 Vitamin C 2mcg 17% Calcium 270mg 15% Iron 17mg 20% Potassium 130mg 2%

Vegan Cake

I Vegan Cake f you are tired or very busy during the week, I recommend you set aside a few hours on the weekends to do your baking. Bake one or two yummy vegan snack recipes to last you the week and freeze them in portions. Find some easy (or gourmet if you wish) vegan cake recipes, muffin recipes, brownie recipes, or slice recipes that look delicious and that you know you will satisfy your snack cravings during the week.

Vegan Health Slice

Once again, if you bake it on the weekends, you will not have to prepare your morning and afternoon tea during the week. There are so many delicious recipes nowadays for vegan health slices. There's an apple-crumble slice, oat and nut slice, dried-fruit slice, blueberry slice, chocolate-brownie slice, and so many more delicious recipes! Why not bake a different vegan piece every weekend? This will keep your vegan snacks from becoming dull. As you can see, your vegan snacks can be speedy and easy to prepare. And it's always an excellent habit to get into to do your vegan baking on the weekend so that your mid-week snacks can be hassle-free!

Spicy Apple Crisp

Ingredients:

8 cooking apples 4 oz. or then again 150 g flour 7 oz. or on the other hand 350 g earthy colored sugar 5 oz. or then again 175 g vegetarian margarine ¼ tablespoon ground cinnamon ¼ tablespoon ground nutmeg Zest of one lemon 1 tablespoon new lemon juice

Directions

: Peel, quarter, and center cooking apples. Cut apple quarters into low cuts and spot them in a bowl. Mix nutmeg and cinnamon. At that point, sprinkle over apples. Sprinkle with lemon skin. Add lemon squeeze and throw to mix. Orchestrate cuts in a huge preparing dish. Make a combination of sugar, flour, and vegetarian margarine in a blending bowl. At that point, put over apples, streamlining it. Spot the word in the broiler. Heat at 370°F, 190°C or gas mark 5 for an hour, until seared and apples are delicate.

Apple Cake

Ingredients:

2 oz. or on the other hand 50 g flour 3 tablespoons heating powder ½ tablespoon of salt 2 tablespoons vegetarian shortening ¼ half quart or 125 ml unsweetened soya milk 4 or 5 apples 4 oz. or then again 110 g sugar 1 tablespoon cinnamon.

Guidelines:

Filter together flour, heating powder, and salt. Add shortening and focus on delicately. Add milk gradually to make delicate batter and blend. Spot on floured board and carry out ½ inch or 1 cm thick. Put into the shallow lubed skillet. Wash, pare, center and cut apples into areas; press them into the mixture. Sprinkle with sugar and residue with cinnamon. Heat at 375°F, 190°C or gas mark 5 for 30 minutes or until apples are delicate and earthy colored. Present with soya cream.

Wholesome Facts

Servings per holder 8 Prep Total 10 min Serving Size 2 Amount for every serving Calories 0% % Daily Value Total Fat 4g 210% Saturated Fat 3g 32% Trans Fat 2g 2% Cholesterol 8% Sodium 300mg 0.2% Total Carbohydrate 20g 50%Dietary Fiber 1g 1% Total Sugar 1g 1% Protein 3g Vitamin C 1mcg 18% Calcium 20mg 1% Iron 8mg 12% Potassium 70mg 21%

Apple Charlotte

Ingredients:

2 lbs. or then again 900 g great cooking apples 4 oz. or on the other hand 50 g almonds (hacked) 2 oz. or on the other hand, 50 g currants and sultanas blended 1 stick cinnamon (around 3 inches or 7 cm long) Juice of ½ a lemon Whole bread (cut meagerly) spread Sugar to taste.

Guidelines:

Pare, center, and cut up the apples. Stew the apples with a teacupful of water and the cinnamon until the apples have become a mash. Eliminate the cinnamon, add sugar, lemon squeeze, the almonds, and the currants and sultanas (recently picked, washed, and dried). Blend all well and permit the combination to cool. Oil a pie-dish and line it with flimsy cuts of meat and potatoes. Then put on it a layer of apple combination, rehash the layers, and get done with amounts of bread and vegetarian margarine. Prepare at 375°F, 190°C or gas mark 5 for 45 minutes.

Vegan Brownie

Ingredients:

1/2 cup non-dairy spread dissolved 5 tablespoons cocoa 1 cup granulated sugar 3 teaspoons Ener-G egg replacer 1/4 cup water 1 teaspoon vanilla 3/4 cup flour 1 teaspoon preparing powder 1/2 teaspoon salt 1/2 cup pecans (discretionary)

Directions:

Warmth broiler to 350°. Set up an 8" x 8" heating skillet with spread or canola oil. Join spread, cocoa, and sugar in an enormous bowl. Blend the egg replacer and water in a blender until foamy. Add to the spread blend with vanilla. Add the flour, heating powder, and salt, and blend thoroughly. Add the pecans whenever wanted. Empty the player into the skillet and spread uniformly. Heat for 40 to 45 minutes, or until a toothpick embedded tells the truth.

Chapter 5: Tips and tricks to stay healthy after 50

Preparation is the key to succeeding in intermittent fasting. When you prepare well, you can be sure to stay in control so that you're not feeling lost and out of place. If you want to reap the benefits of intermittent fasting quickly, you must be keen to make the right move when getting into this practice. Your body is accustomed to eating after 2-3 hours; therefore, you need to immerse yourself into fasting systematically. Although this sounds simple in principle, it's actually not easy when you start out. However, when you take caution and come up with a good plan, you'll have a smooth transition that will contribute to your intermittent fasting quest's success. Here are some warnings you can consider while making the transition to intermittent fasting:

Transition slowly

It's okay to be ambitious about going without food for several hours. However, as you're starting out, you need to be careful not to be too ambitious by immersing yourself in intermittent fasting that requires you to fast for extended periods. It's advisable to consider starting with the simpler intermittent fasting protocols and advance to the comprehensive protocols over time. If anything, you gained the weight you're trying to shed off after a long time, so don't expect to lose weight overnight. For instance, you can start with the 12:12 intermittent fasting protocol where you have a fasting window of 12 hours to advancing on to 16:8, which lets you fast for 16 hours and eat for 8 hours. You can even take a break after a couple of days or weeks before attempting again. The trick is to make sure that you're adding on another day every week until you're able to stick to your intermittent fasting plan. Only then can you consider trying intermittent fasting protocols that require you to fast for extended periods of between 18 and 24 hours, like 5:2 or warrior, depending on how comfortable you're. Don't hesitate to tailor the fasting protocol to your preference, even if it means not doing it every day.

Take your schedule into account.

It's essential to keep your schedule in mind while planning for the intermittent fasting protocol that's right for you. Your choice of an intermittent fasting protocol should not be influenced by peer pressure instead of suitable for you concerning your schedule. Don't go for an extreme plan in the beginning just because your friends are doing it. Suppose there's no way you can have your meals within an 8-hour window because your schedule is erratic. In that case, the LeanGains 16:8 protocol is not appropriate for you. However, if you are sure you can't go for 24 hours without food, then this intermittent plan might be the most suitable for you. Ultimately, you must think about your schedule, preferences. If the project affects the other people, you live with before deciding what is best for you. This will make your transition to intermittent fasting smooth.

Don't start intermittent fasting alongside a new diet.

If your goal is to lose weight and be interested in taking on a new diet like a low-calorie diet or keto, make sure you're not starting it alongside intermittent fasting. This is because it takes time for your body to adjust to your diet's new meals and foods. Moreover, whether you're cutting down on meat on your vegetarian diet or you're simply reducing your carbs dramatically, it will have a significant effect on your body when combined with intermittent fasting. Therefore, to succeed with intermittent fasting, make sure that you stick to your diet for up to two weeks before adding intermittent fasting. This way, you will have a great understanding of your body, hence a smooth transition.

Eliminate snacks.

Snacks refer to anything that will add empty calories to your system and cause cravings. Before beginning intermittent fasting, make sure you prepare your body to stay without food for more extended periods than usual. The first step towards this is eliminating snacks. Although not evident, snacks are your biggest enemies because they're not nutritious; instead, they're only full of salt, sugar, flours, and refined oil. Thus, you must learn to avoid them to stay in shape. Snacks often cause your blood sugar levels to spike while loading your system with empty calories and provide very little to your gut. Make sure you eliminate snacks from your routine. You also need to avoid carbonated beverages that add empty calories and are full of sugar.

Most importantly, keep in mind that intermittent fasting is not based on restricting your calorie intake, so you can consume calories within a reasonable limit. Somewhat, your calorie intake will automatically reduce since your eating windows are short. Remember, intermittent fasting is based on when you eat and not what you eat. One of the best ways to avoid processed foods is staying away from foods served at fast-food chains, including salads with various dressings. Instead, make it a habit to cook your own food. This will ensure you're only eating healthy food.

Stay true to your purpose.

There's definitely a reason why you're getting into intermittent fasting. Staying true to this reason is the only way you'll stay grounded to the cause. Therefore, make sure you have defined the reason why you're going into fasting. This may be losing weight; fasting will reduce the level of hormones like insulin while increasing the human growth hormone and norepinephrine that make the stored body fat more accessible, making it possible for you to burn fat and effectively lose weight. Fasting also helps in the prevention of heart disease, diabetes, as well as reduce inflammation. Most importantly, fasting will also offer protection against cancer, Alzheimer's while increasing longevity.

Face your fears

It's normal to feel nervous and even harbor doubts before beginning intermittent fasting, mainly because we have been cultured to believe that breakfast is the most important meal of the day. However, you need to know that when unaddressed, these worries can cause you to stop. Therefore, face them. It's important to know that breakfast is a neutral meal; hence can be skipped. In fact, the reality is that skipping breakfast will not make you gain weight while eating breakfast will not rave up your metabolism. You also need to keep in mind that fasting will increase your metabolic rate and help you lose weight while retaining more muscle.

Begin with 3 meals.

 Intermittent fasting is all about a total lifestyle change. Therefore, you need to start by taking three meals. This may be surprising, and you may be wondering whether the fact that you're already skipping a meal means you are doing intermittent fasting. Well, the answer is no. Here's why; while you don't have time to consume three meals on any given day, you somewhat take improper meals in the day. This kind of munching counts for intermittent fasting. Thus, we must consider starting off with a balanced breakfast, eat moderate lunch, and finish with a light dinner. When you get to a point where you can sustain without difficulty with the three meals, you'll be ready to move on to intermittent fasting.

Be consistent with your intermittent fasting protocol.

 You will likely be excited to make a change and transition to the following intermittent fasting protocol after some time. This is especially the case when you begin seeing results. Even then, you must remember that intermittent fasting mustn't be rushed. Make sure you stay on a single fasting protocol for at least two weeks before moving on to the next. Keep in mind that each of the intermittent fasting protocols presents its own unique results and advantages. Only when you get comfortable should you consider moving on to the next one.

No fasting protocol is superior.

It's a common misconception that you can only get better results when you go for a stricter regimen. While there's some degree of truth in this belief, it's essential to focus on individual capacity. Everyone has their unique capabilities, thus imitating someone else is utterly meaningless. Some people may post impressive results with a 12-hour fasting protocol. In contrast, for others, it will take another protocol to experience similar products. So, don't go for the toughest protocol but instead find a protocol that suits you.

Focus on eating healthy eating.

One of the things you're likely to ignore when starting intermittent fasting is the quality of food you're eating. Although your fast will generally involve cutting down on the number of calories you're consuming, it's equally important to be deliberate about your food choices. More specifically, focus on healthy eating, especially if you're aiming to make this a lifestyle. While you can eat unhealthy food while doing intermittent fasting, eating healthy foods contribute towards living a long and healthy life. Therefore, be sure to include fruits, nuts, vegetables, healthy fats, and lean proteins in your diet.

Know when to quit.

It is essential that you're flexible and adapts to your changing needs. For instance, if your plan is to fast for 16 hours, but you begin feeling tired, you might as well shorten your day. You may also be working out, but you generally feel you donat have enough energy; this is also a reason to break your fast early. You shouldn't aim to be perfect at the expense of your well-being. Suppose you begin feeling sick during your fasting window. In that case, it's better to be consistent than to be perfect.

Keep it simple.

Unlike many other diets designed to help in losing weight, intermittent fasting doesn't require you to deviate from your usual meals to some sophisticated menus. Therefore, aim at eating your regular meals during your eating window. However, you can also consider combining your intermittent fasting regimen with a low carb, high-fat diet comprising whole natural foods. Get enough rest. Fasting, by itself, is not enough if you want to embrace a healthy lifestyle. Make sure you're also getting enough sleep. Your body requires rest to be able to carry out some of the essential functions. Therefore, don't work at night unless it's necessary. We aren't wired as other nocturnal beings; thus, we need to follow through with our circadian rhythm. When you get sound sleep at night, no doubt your body will be able to fight off the weight in a better way even as your stress and cholesterol levels improve. If anything, intermittent fasting puts emphasis on giving the body adequate sleep. Make sure you plan your day so that you free up some time for good sleep. Most importantly, make sure you rest more when you fast for extended periods.

Practice perseverance

Unfortunately, most people that have a problem with their weight are also impatient. This is probably because they're already under pressure to lose weight, yet it's just not happening. Moreover, most people trying to lose weight have already tried other ways of shedding excess fat unsuccessfully and looking for quick results. Unfortunately, intermittent fasting is not an overnight success. It takes time and consistency before you can see the results. You must be ready to see the change happen after a while since you're correcting problems/weight accumulated over the years. Don't lose hope in the process because by quitting, you can't tell whether you had made any progress. You can stall hunger by laughing, running, talking to friends, or engaging in activities that delay needing.

Hydrate during fasting

It's essential always to make sure you're drinking up enough during intermittent fasting. Yet, it's common to find beginners thinking that they should not consume anything during the fasting window. This is wrong because intermittent fasting allows you to take water, tea, or coffee as long as you don't use any cream, milk, or sugar. Staying hydrated is essential in extending your satiety; thus, drinking water will help you get rid of that feeling of hunger.

Manage your fasting time properly.

It's common for people to mismanage time during the fasting window, just as is with our regular schedules. You need to know that not managing your fasting time well is likely to cause distress. This can make your journey of losing weight painful and difficult. Stop thinking about food the entire time you're in the fasted state. This will create problems since your gut will be confused. You can manage your fasting time by staying busy while ensuring that you're engaged until the last leg of your fasting window. When you're idle, likely, you'll only be thinking about food. Think about ways of putting off hunger. After all, our bodies have ample energy reserves that can run without food for a long time.

Don't rush the process.

We all want quick results, but you have to follow through with the process with intermittent fasting. Don't attempt to make short jumps because the body doesn't work this way. The transition process of your body is relatively slow. Thus, you need to allow more time to adjust to the change that comes with intermittent fasting. To succeed with each of these processes, make sure you stay at every stage for some time. This gives your body time to adjust to the changes. Remember, you're trying to change habits that are decades old, so you need to be patient to make your body adjust to the process. The other thing you must remember is that fasting is different in men and women. While a man's system is rugged and doesn't get to be affected by extended fasting periods, fasting can affect a woman's health adversely; hence, it takes time to normalize—accordingly, the need to start small and advance with time.

Have realistic expectations.

It's okay to have a goal and dreams about your weight loss goals. Even then, make sure that you're grounded in reality. This is an excellent place to start as you can accept facts and avoid lots of disappointments. Having unrealistic expectations often contributes to the failure to recognize the benefits you derive from the process. For instance, if your goal is losing weight, you must really think about the amount of time you'll put into fasting and your overall commitment. Not taking all the relevant factors into consideration will leave you feeling frustrated and difficult to achieve the results you desire.

Determine how long you want to fast/create a routine.

Since intermittent fasting is more of a pattern of eating than a diet fad, you can only get the best results when you follow it in routine. This means that you will not get the results if you're just practicing fasting in an unstructured way. If anything, irregularly doing intermittent fasting will not yield any results; instead, it'll leave you feeling hungry. Your gut releases the hunger hormone with so much accuracy. As such, the soul can sense the time when you eat so that you think gurgling in your stomach around precisely the same time the next day. This means that if you're keeping a 14-hour fast regularly, you'll notice you feel hungry hunger just about the time you need to break your fast. This means that if you don't keep a regular routine, then this will not happen. Making intermittent fasting a usual way will help you get over the hassle of being too conscious. After a while, this would be part of your lifestyle hence easy to follow.

Don't be greedy when it's time to breaking your fast

Food is the fascinating thing you can encounter when you've been deprived of it for long hours. It's actually tempting. You need to make sure that you don't get greedy when breaking your fast, somewhat correctly, get off the quick. The biggest mistake you can make is eating a lot as it can lead to various problems, among them poor digestion. Your gut can be dry after long periods of fasting. Thus, stuffing it with heavy food can result in problems. When breaking your fast, start with liquid food, slowly transitioning to semi-solid and finally solid foods. You also need to check the quantity of food that you eat because the brain takes time to decode the leptin signals that you're full. When the brain finally signals, you're full, you'll have to overeat. This means that you need to eat slowly so that your brain has enough time to determine your satiety levels. Alternatively, stop eating when you're at 80% complete, after which you're unlikely to feel hungry again. You only require a few calories during intermittent fasting because your body is running on just a few calories or no food at all for a more extended period than usual. This can result in having a hangover initially. You can train your body to come with the stress linked to food deprivation to get used to staying for long without food. If you realize that you can't cope with your intermittent fasting plan, you can consider switching to another plan. You might have chosen a program that is not suitable for your needs or lifestyle. Don't be discouraged if one method doesn't work. Instead, make sure you work towards finding the proper fasting protocol that you'll be comfortable with while getting the results you need. By transitioning into intermittent slowly, you're giving your body a chance to self-regulate and gradually adapt to your changing eating pattern. It also diminishes or avoids early transition symptoms that include dry mouth, insomnia, and digestive changes.

Chapter 6: FAQ About intermittent fasting

Why am I not losing fat faster, like other people are?

Intermittent fasting, not getting more fit If you're not shedding pounds—regardless of remaining inside your calorie needs—at that point, it's an ideal opportunity to see serving sizes. It's entirely expected to err the amount you're really eating, which prompts devouring a more significant number of calories than you might suspect. This is especially evident with calorie-thick food sources like cheddar.

Can I have a cheat meal?

Permit yourself some cheat suppers. Irregular fasting can get monotonous throughout a significant period. Permit yourself to have up to three cheat suppers a month yet be mindful so as not to try too hard.

Can I have coffee?

Indeed, you can drink plain, dark espresso during discontinuous fasting. Most sans calorie drinks are protected to burn-through during irregular fasting. However, a few dietitians don't suggest diet drinks with counterfeit sugars.

Do I have to eat low carb?

The best an ideal opportunity to eat carbs when you practice discontinuous fasting. Irregular fasting is eating and fasting during specific windows of time. On the off chance that you follow this kind of eating design, Patton says it's OK to eat carbs all through your whole window — regardless of whether your objective is weight reduction or in case you're diabetic or pre-diabetic.

Should I exercise in the fasted state?

One hypothesis is that practicing in an abstained state may help consume fat. Lowden clarifies that the body needs sugar or some kind of energy to perform well while working out. Ordinarily, the power comes from sugar particles, which are put away as glycogen in the liver. "Assuming you begin working out, you're bound to exhaust those stores, and your body must choose the option to go into a more anaerobic breakdown to give you the energy you need," she says. Rather than consuming sugars that aren't accessible, your body is compelled to finish another fuel source: fat.

However, you might not have sufficient energy to practice as seriously as you regularly would. "Pinnacle execution or in any event, feeling better while practicing it's a lot simpler to do on the off chance that you eat."

Why should one start intermittent fasting?

Other than weight reduction, are there different advantages to discontinuous fasting? Notwithstanding decreased bodyweight, this fasting can help lower cholesterol, improve glucose control, diminish liver fat and improve the circulatory strain. Patients reveal to me they have expanded perseverance, better engine coordination, and improved rest.

Will intermittent fasting affect one's metabolism?

Numerous individuals accept that skipping dinners will make your body adjust by bringing its metabolic rate down to save energy. It's grounded that significant stretches without food can cause a drop in indigestion. In any case, considers have shown that fasting for brief periods can really build your digestion, not back it off. One investigation in 11 solid men tracked down that a 3-day quick really expanded their digestion by an impressive 14 percent. This increment is believed to be because of the ascent in the chemical norepinephrine, which advances fat consumption.

Chapter 7: Conclusion

Thank you for making it through to the end of Intermittent Fasting for Women; let's hope it was informative and able to provide you with all of the tools you need to achieve your goals, whatever they may be. The next step is to take action that will usher you into a new level of wellness. If you still need help getting started, you are likely to get better results by evaluating your current schedule before you can select an appropriate intermittent fasting plan that is realistic, to begin with. Remember, you'll not be doing this to please anyone but for your own benefit. Intermittent fasting is an excellent concept of scheduling your mealtimes, not just for weight loss but also for living holistically. It gives you access to numerous health benefits.

What's more? Unlike many weight-loss diets that are restrictive, expensive, and offer minimal results, intermittent fasting is free and easy to follow through. You simply need to change your eating pattern to have periods of fasting followed by periods of feasting. This book is primarily a great resource to help you through your journey in carving a new lifestyle. Remember, you don't have to change your way of living but instead embrace the new way of feeding to suit your way of living. In fact, you can still carry on with your exercise routine even though you may have to tailor it to your current situation in terms of when you eat and how intense your workout is. What are you waiting for? Go ahead and start preparing for your intermittent fasting experience to tap into its benefits. Use the information you have acquired in this book as a springboard to design and transform your life.

My goal for this guide was to put very complex and technical concepts most simply, to make them readable for everyone. I accurately selected what I believe are the most valuable and influential pieces of advice for you to do what I mentioned above. In my 30 years+ of professional experience, I've had the fantastic chance to deal with thousands of people of all ages, gender, and personality. It inevitably has some reflections on my writings. I don't like to call myself an author, yet I have to admit that I learned a lot while writing books over the past few years. In fact, what I got from those past publications was validation from readers who enjoyed my work and encouraged me to keep writing. I always value the opinion of readers and take into account criticism as well. I believe that reviews are a great way to give someone credit for the work done, and I love reading them all the time. However, I hope I accomplished at least the goal I had in my mind - which was to provide you precious information about intermittent fasting, based on scientific studies as well as my own experience, and, most importantly, I hope you learned something new and will act on it to change your life.

Thank you for reading This book.

If you enjoyed it, please visit the site where you purchased it and write a brief review. Your feedback is important to me and will help other readers decide whether to read the book too.

Thank you!   **Angela D. Cook**

CPSIA information can be obtained
at www.ICGtesting.com
Printed in the USA
BVHW050316080521
606757BV00009B/1187